Workbook
BEING A
NURSING ASSISTANT

BRADY

Workbook

BEING A
NURSING ASSISTANT

SEVENTH EDITION

JoLynn Pullium, MS, RN, CPHQ

Rose B. Schniedman, CNA, MSEd, BSN, RN

Susan S. Lambert, MAEd

Barbara R. Wander, BSN, RN

American Hospital Association

Francie Wolgin

BRADY
Prentice Hall
Upper Saddle River, New Jersey 07458
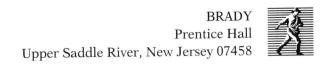

Publisher: *Susan Katz*
Marketing Manager: *Judy Streger*
Acquisitions Editor: *Barbara Krawiec*
Managing Development Editor: *Marilyn Meserve*
Editorial Assistant: *Louise Fullam*
Director of Manufacturing & Production: *Bruce Johnson*
Managing Production Editor: *Patrick Walsh*
Senior Production Manager: *Ilene Sanford*
Editorial/Composition/Production/Design Supervision:
  Elm Street Publishing Services, Inc.
Cover Design: *Bruce Kenselaar*
Cover Photographs: *Michal Heron*
Managing Photography Editor: *Michal Heron*
Printing and Binding: *Banta Printing Company*

ISBN 0-89303-021-X

PRENTICE HALL INTERNATIONAL (UK) LIMITED, *London*
PRENTICE HALL OF AUSTRALIA PTY. LIMITED, *Sydney*
PRENTICE HALL OF CANADA INC., *Toronto*
PRENTICE HALL OF HISPANOAMERICANA, S.A., *Mexico*
PRENTICE HALL OF INDIA PRIVATE LIMITED, *New Delhi*
PRENTICE HALL OF JAPAN, INC., *Tokyo*
SIMON & SCHUSTER ASIA PTE. LTD., *Singapore*
EDITORA PRENTICE HALL DO BRASIL, LTDA., *Rio de Janeiro*

Note on Gender Usage

The English language has historically given
preference to the male gender. Among many
words, the pronouns, "he" and "his," are commonly used to describe both genders. The
male pronouns still predominate our speech,
however, in this workbook "he" and "she" have
been used interchangeably when referring to
the Nursing Assistant and/or the patient. The
repeated use of "he or she" is not proper in
long manuscript, and the use of "he or she" is
not correct in all cases. The authors have
made a great effort to treat the two genders
equally. Throughout the workbook, solely for
the purpose of brevity, male pronouns and
female pronouns are often used to describe
both males and females. This is not intended
to offend any reader of the female or male
gender.

Notice of Intent

The procedures described in the textbook and
this workbook are based on consultation with
nursing authorities. To the best of the authors'
knowledge, these procedures reflect currently
accepted clinical practice; however, they cannot be considered absolute recommendations.
For individual application, the policies and
procedures of the institution or agency where
the Nursing Assistant is employed must be
reviewed and followed. The authors of the textbook, and of the supplements written specifi-
cally to go with it, disclaim responsibility for
any adverse effects resulting directly or indi-
rectly from the suggested procedures and
theory, from any undetected errors, or from
the reader's misunderstanding of the text. It is
the reader's responsibility to stay informed of
any new changes or recommendations made
by his or her employing health care institution
or agency.

If when reading this workbook you find an
error, have an idea for how to improve it, or
simply want to share your comments with us,
please send your letter to the authors at

Brady Marketing Department
c/o Judy Streger
Prentice Hall
One Lake Street
Upper Saddle River, NJ 07458

▶ Contents

1 The Health Care System 1

2 Your Role as a Nursing Assistant 9

3 Communication Skills 15

4 Patients, Residents, and Clients 25

5 Infection Control 33

6 Safety 41

7 Body Mechanics: Positioning, Moving, and Transporting Patients 47

8 Admitting, Transferring, and Discharging a Patient 63

9 The Patient's Environment 69

10 Bedmaking 75

11 Home Health Care 79

12 Personal Care of the Patient 87

13 Emergency Care 93

14 The Human Body 99

15 Growth and Development 105

16 The Musculoskeletal System and Related Care 109

17 The Integumentary System and Related Care 117

18 The Circulatory and Respiratory Systems and Related Care 123

19 Measuring Vital Signs 133

20 The Gastrointestinal System and Related Care 147

21 Nutrition for the Patient 155

22 The Urinary System and Related Care 163

23 Specimen Collection 171

24 The Endocrine System and Related Care of Diabetics 177

25 The Reproductive System and Related Care 185

26 The Nervous System and Related Care 193

27 Warm and Cold Applications 199

28 Care of the Surgical Patient 205

29 Special Procedures 215

30 Other Patients with Special Needs 219

31 Neonatal and Pediatric Care 225

32 The Older Adult Patient and Long-Term Care 231

33 Rehabilitation and Return to Self-Care 237

34   The Terminally Ill Patient and Postmortem Care   245

35   Beginning Your Career as a Nursing Assistant   253

Appendix: Medical Terms, Abbreviations, and Specialties   259

▶ Introduction

This workbook has been written to motivate interest, to instruct, to evaluate, and to involve you, the student, actively in the learning process. We ask you to:

- Locate, recall, and recognize information
- Change information into different forms, such as from pictures to words
- Discover relationships and facts, definitions, rules, procedures, and skills
- Find solutions to lifelike situations
- Learn by doing

A variety of exercises from word searches to multiple choice questions have been included in an effort to meet your individual learning needs and to provide an effective learning experience that is compatible with your learning style. The knowledge and skill you gain will help you face the new experiences on the job as a nursing assistant.

This workbook is not intended to be used alone. It is totally dependent and coordinated with the textbook, *Being a Nursing Assistant, Seventh Edition.* It is planned to guide you through the textbook, and it is absolutely essential that you read the textbook as you do each assignment. If you read something that puzzles you, ask your instructor to explain it.

This is not a book of tests. We encourage you to keep your textbook open as you do each assignment. The questions in this workbook were not written to stump, trick, or fool you. They were written to help you learn to do the nursing tasks and procedures you will be reading about and studying in your textbook.

You can also use the workbook to review your classroom and clinical learning experiences. By completing these assignments, you can fix the procedures and key ideas firmly in your mind. If you are willing to be an active participant in the learning experiences, this workbook can help you with key terms and can be an effective learning tool.

The more you read, review, and practice, the easier it will be for you to take the step from being a student to being a nursing assistant.

THE HEALTH CARE SYSTEM

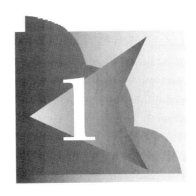

The following exercises will assist you to apply what you have read in Chapter 1, "The Health Care System." For each exercise, read the objective and use information you have read in Chapter 1 to answer the questions, complete the sentences, or label the diagrams.

EXERCISE 1-1

Objective: To recognize and correctly spell words related to the health care system.

Directions: Unscramble the words in the Word List at the left. Then circle these same words in the Word Search at the right.

Word List

1. RDG _____ DRG's
2. AANMDGE RAEC _____ Managed care
3. AETM _____ Team
4. IMRPRYA _____ Primary
5. AKST _____ Tast
6. SPRUEVRIOS _____ Supervisor
7. TAIPNET OCFSDUE _____ patient Focused
8. SRGIETEEDR ESRUN _____ Registered nurse

Word Search

L	E	S	I	T	K	X	S	H	K	L	F	Q	Y	K
P	S	B	Q	A	W	Z	F	W	U	D	G	C	P	Z
A	R	U	O	V	B	U	D	I	O	P	N	I	W	X
T	U	T	A	G	S	C	R	H	A	R	G	N	E	Y
I	N	E	I	L	Y	E	A	C	Q	I	B	Y	O	T
E	D	A	B	F	T	I	G	F	N	M	S	K	L	U
N	E	M	A	N	A	G	E	D	C	A	R	E	I	K
T	R	A	B	E	S	O	N	R	U	R	D	P	G	Q
F	E	H	I	M	K	J	A	G	N	Y	S	E	M	X
O	T	K	D	T	R	H	K	D	B	L	C	J	E	R
C	S	R	O	S	I	V	R	E	P	U	S	S	N	I
U	I	G	F	G	X	I	M	P	A	Y	T	O	H	O
S	G	L	B	I	C	P	E	R	O	I	A	C	J	U
E	E	W	M	O	V	O	T	Y	M	U	V	T	X	D
D	R	N	C	P	S	A	W	J	H	E	Y	I	Z	Z
C	B	V	A	E	F	Z	X	A	W	Q	B	M	X	A
Y	R	T	B	D	L	K	U	O	J	P	N	Z	G	W
Z	I	K	O	E	B	Z	H	Z	E	C	V	J	C	H
X	F	M	Q	R	L	T	Y	H	A	Y	K	I	S	E

EXERCISE 1-2

Objective: To apply what you have learned about the health care system and the nursing assistant.

Directions: Circle the letter next to the statement that best completes the sentence or describes the sentence as true or false. If the sentence is false, draw a line through the incorrect part of the sentence and write the correction on the blank line.

1. Factors directly affecting the health care system are all of the following *except*
    A. government legislation.
    B. an aging population.
    C. managed care.
    D. floral deliveries.

2. The nursing assistant in his role is able to directly contribute to the health care system if he can effectively participate in
    A. patient-focused care.
    B. the team approach.
    C. cost-effective quality care.
    D. all of the above.

3. It is important to understand the organizational structure of the facility you work at because
    A. knowing this will help you to be more successful in your role.
    B. it might be asked on a test.
    C. you will get paid more for knowing this.
    D. you want to impress your friends.

4. At the center of the multidisciplinary team approach is the
    A. nurse.
    B. nursing assistant.
    C. doctor.
    D. patient.

5. Patient-focused care means that the patient's needs are considered last when planning individualized care.
    A. True
    B. False
    Correct Answer: _FiRST_____

6. Preventing disease is an important aspect of the _____ system.
    A. postal
    B. digestive
    C. infective
    D. health care

7. Because the health care system is continually changing, the successful nursing assistant will be looking for opportunities to
    A. work fewer hours.
    B. learn new skills to keep up with these changes.
    C. remain the same, because it always worked in the past.
    D. do his best to resist change.

8. Patients and family are becoming more involved with
    A. self-care.
    B. your-care.
    C. unknown-care.
    D. rapid-care.

9. DRG stands for
    A. divisional regulated growth.
    B. diagnostic rules and groups.
    C. diagnosis-related groups.
    D. diagonally related growth.

10. To be effective, health care must go beyond the care provided in the hospital to consider the health needs of the community.
    A. True
    B. False
    Correct Answer: _____

11. CPT–4 stands for
    A. Cost-Preventive Treatment–4th edition.
    B. Currently-Posted Trials–4th edition.
    C. Collective Procedural Terminology–4th edition.
    D. Current Procedural Terminology–4th edition.

12. The goal of quality care is to improve the individual's health status as much as possible.
    A. True
    B. False
    Correct Answer: _____

13. The goal of managed care is to balance quality care, cost, and access.
    A. True
    B. False
    Correct Answer: _____

14. Health care financing refers to _____, who pay for hospital visits, clinic visits, prescription medications, home care visits, hospice care, and other health care services.
    A. insurance companies
    B. managed care entities
    C. individuals
    D. all of the above

15. Health care delivery refers to _____, who provide health care services to patients.
    A. nursing assistants, doctors, nurses, therapists
    B. hospitals, clinics, surgical centers
    C. rehabilitation centers, hospices, home care agencies
    D. all of the above

16. There are several different kinds of nursing care team structures, but a common element is
    A. a nurse accountable for the patient's nursing care.
    B. a nursing assistant as part of the team.
    C. fee-for-service payment.
    D. a doctor performing nursing tasks.

17. The nursing assistant will most likely function on all of the following *except* the
    A. Functional Nursing Team Model.
    B. Team Nursing Model.
    C. Patient-focused Care Model.
    D. Primary Nursing Model.

18. No matter what team the nursing assistant works on, the most important element of his success is
    A. to discuss his assignments with the patient.
    B. to discuss his assignment and any questions he may have with his immediate supervisor.
    C. to discuss everything with the team.
    D. to discuss the patients he cares for with his friends.

19. Based on the _____, nursing assistants must complete an approved training program before working in skilled nursing facilities and nursing homes.
    A. Omnibus Budget Reconciliation Act (OBRA) of 1987
    B. direction of the Skilled Nursing Act
    C. American Nursing Home Authority
    D. TEFRA of 1982

EXERCISE 1-3

Objective: To apply what you have learned about organizational structures and the nursing assistant's "chain of command."

Directions: Label the blank spaces on the organizational chart in Figure 1-1. Place the words from the Word List below in the proper order on the diagram.

Word List

Board of Directors 1
VP of Operations 3
Nurse Managers 5

Staff Nurses 6
LPNs 7
President 2

Director of Nurses 4
Nursing Assistants 8

FIGURE 1-1

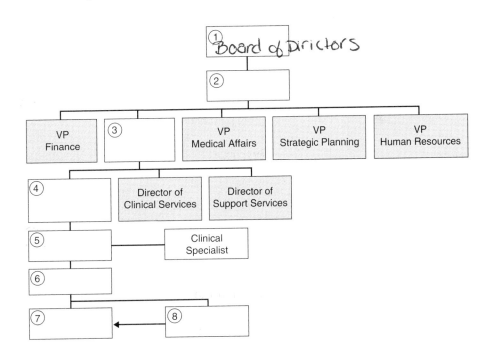

EXERCISE 1-4

Objective: To apply what you have learned about the multidisciplinary patient care team.

Directions: Label the multidisciplinary patient care team diagram in Figure 1-2 with the correct words from the Word List below. Choose from the list only those who are part of this team.

Word List

Clergy	Pharmacist	~~Beautician~~	Nursing Assistant ✓
Patient	~~Veterinarian~~	Physician ✓	Speech Therapist
~~Manicurist~~	Family ✓	Social Worker	~~Coach~~
Dentist ✓	~~Engineer~~	~~Pilot~~	Registered Nurse ✓

FIGURE 1-2

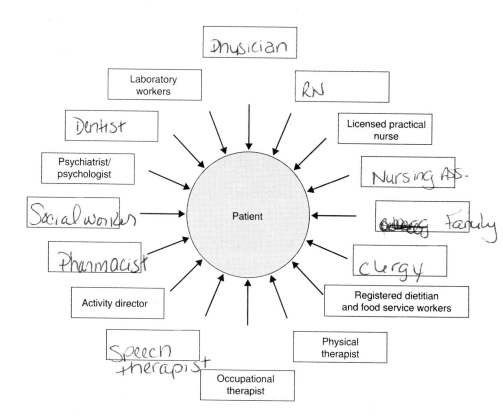

EXERCISE 1-5

Objective: To recognize the definitions of words related to the health care system.

Directions: Place the letter of the correct definition next to the matching word from the Word List.

<table>
<tr><th colspan="2">Word List</th><th>Definitions</th></tr>
<tr><td>I</td><td>1. nurse</td><td>A. A physician's determination of a patient's disease or condition.</td></tr>
<tr><td>E</td><td>2. hospice</td><td>B. Diagnostically related groups of patients.</td></tr>
<tr><td>A</td><td>3. diagnosis</td><td>C. A method of organizing the health care team in which the head nurse assigns and directs all patient care responsibilities for the nursing staff.</td></tr>
<tr><td>B</td><td>4. DRGs</td><td>D. Hospital, hospice, nursing home, convalescent home, or clinic where health care services are provided both on an inpatient and outpatient basis.</td></tr>
<tr><td>H</td><td>5. multidisciplinary team</td><td>E. An extended, or long term, care facility that provides health care services to terminally ill patients and their families.</td></tr>
<tr><td>C</td><td>6. functional nursing</td><td>F. A short term, or emergency, care facility that provides health care services to patients.</td></tr>
<tr><td>D</td><td>7. health care institution</td><td>G. An individual responsible for providing direction, critiquing performance, and giving feedback related to that performance.</td></tr>
<tr><td>G</td><td>8. immediate supervisor</td><td>H. A team of professionals and nonprofessionals from different disciplines that plans and implements patient-focused care.</td></tr>
<tr><td>F</td><td>9. hospital</td><td>I. A person educated and trained to provide health care for people, working with physicians and other health care team members; licensed as RNs and LPNs.</td></tr>
<tr><td>N</td><td>10. managed care</td><td>J. A person who helps the registered nurse to care for patients.</td></tr>
<tr><td>Q</td><td>11. team nursing</td><td>K. The RN leader responsible for the care delivery, personnel supervision, and operating budget of a unit, area, or facility.</td></tr>
<tr><td>P</td><td>12. team leader</td><td>L. A care delivery model in which multidisciplinary teams plan and implement care based on the patient's individual needs.</td></tr>
<tr><td>O</td><td>13. task oriented</td><td>M. A patient-oriented method of organizing the health care team in which the professional registered nurses are responsible and accountable for the entire nursing care of the patient.</td></tr>
</table>

works under a RN or LPN

_K_ 14. nurse manager

_M_ 15. primary nursing

_J_ 16. nursing assistant

_L_ 17. patient-focused
care

N. Care provided under a wide variety of pre-payment agreements, negotiated contracts and discounts, agreements for prior service authorization or approval, and performance audits.

O. Nursing care that is arranged according to what must be done.

P. The nurse responsible for one area of a nursing unit, including patient care assignments.

Q. A task-oriented method of organizing the health care team in which the team leader gives patient care assignments to each team member.

YOUR ROLE AS A NURSING ASSISTANT

The following exercises will assist you to apply what you have read in Chapter 2, "Your Role as a Nursing Assistant." For each exercise, read the objective and use information you have read in Chapter 2 to answer the questions, complete the sentences, or label the diagrams.

EXERCISE 2-1

Objective: To apply what you have learned about personal hygiene and appearance.

Directions: Look carefully at the pictures in Figure 2-1. Choose the number of the sentence on the Personal Hygiene List that indicates the correct personal grooming rule you need to practice on a daily basis. Label the item in Figure 2-1 with the correctly matching number.

Personal Hygiene List

1. Dress properly and neatly. Follow the dress code of the health care institution where you work.
2. Use good personal hygiene, bathing or showering daily.
3. Keep your mouth and teeth clean and in good condition.
4. Keep your hair clean and neatly combed. Long hair should be braided, pulled back, or pinned up.
5. Keep your nails short and clean. Wear only clear nail polish, if any.
6. Wear no or very little makeup.
7. Try to be completely free of odor. Do not use heavy perfume, scented sprays, or heavy shaving lotion. Use an unscented deodorant.
8. Get plenty of sleep. Be alert when you come to work.
9. Keep your body fit; do daily exercises.
10. Wear clean clothes every day.
11. Wear comfortable, low-heeled, enclosed shoes with nonskid soles and heels.
12. Keep your shoes polished and the laces clean.

13. Repair rips and hems and replace missing buttons on your clothing.
14. Eat a well-balanced diet every day.
15. Always wear your name pin and institutional badge.
16. Always wear a wristwatch with a second hand.
17. Always carry a pen and a pad of paper.

FIGURE 2-1

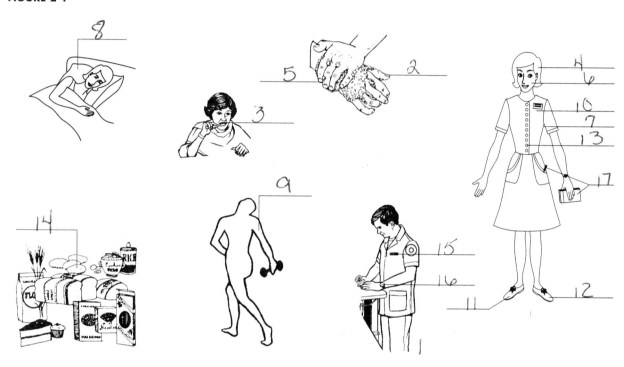

EXERCISE 2-2

Objective: To be able to recognize important concepts of work organization, ethics, work rules, staff relationships, and the legal requirements of patient care.

Directions: Place the correct letters next to the closest matching phrase. There may be more than one correct answer.

> WO = work organization   WR = work rules
> LR = legal requirements   SR = staff relationships
> E = ethics

LR 1. The Patient's Bill of Rights
WR 2. Never discuss your personal problems with patients.
WR 3. Do not waste or destroy supplies or equipment.
E 4. Check the patient's ID bracelet for accuracy.
WO 5. Prioritize your work.
LR 6. Understand how the law affects you and your patient.
E 7. Dependability means more than coming to work on time every day.
SR 8. Work to be a good team member.

_NB_ 9. Be ready to adjust quickly to new situations.

_LR_ 10. Know the laws of your particular state.

_LR_ 11. Civil rights must be guaranteed to all citizens.

_LR_ 12. Good Samaritan laws protect you if you act in good faith during emergencies.

_LR / NR_ 13. Patient confidentiality must be protected.

_LR_ 14. Standards of care are based on laws, administrative policy, and guidelines.

_SR / NR_ 15. Report all complaints from patients and visitors to the immediate supervisor.

_SR_ 16. Volunteer to assist co-workers when you can.

_E_ 17. Respect the right of all patients to have beliefs and opinions different from yours.

_NO_ 18. New needs and unexpected situations may arise, requiring you to adjust your priorities.

_NR_ 19. Perform only procedures that you have been educated to do.

_NO_ 20. Make a written list of your assignments. Review or change the list as you prioritize your work, and check off each item as it is completed.

EXERCISE 2-3

Objective: To apply principles of ethical behavior to challenging situations in which you may be involved.

Directions: Next to each Practice Description, write the number of the correct response.

Practice Description

_3_ A. A patient offers you a tip.

_5_ B. A patient inquires about another patient across the hall.

_4_ C. The patient's ID bracelet is on the bedside stand.

_2_ D. You discover that Mrs. Chang, who is on a low-salt diet, has eaten all of her lunch from a regular diet tray, which you gave her earlier by mistake.

_1_ E. You have a headache, and nothing seems to be going the way it should today.

Response

1. Refrain from sharing your problems as you provide care for others.

2. You notify your immediate supervisor at once.

3. You say, "No, thank you," and pleasantly explain that it is against written policy to accept.

4. You follow the policy of your institution to provide the patient with a new ID band.

5. You give no information about the patient, but you do explain the institution's policy on confidentiality.

EXERCISE 2-4

Objective: To apply what you have learned about your role as a nursing assistant.

Directions: Circle the letter next to the statement that best completes the sentence or describes the sentence as true or false. If the sentence is false, draw a line through the incorrect part of the sentence and write the correction on the blank line.

1. Making false or damaging statements about another person is
   A. known as defamation of character.
   B. known as a good standard of care.
   C. a breach of duty.
   D. a way to strengthen a relationship.

2. Patients have the right to refuse care, even if ~~they are not conscious.~~
   A. True
   B. False
   Correct Answer: _If they are conscious_

3. Leaving your patients without permission or without notifying the immediate supervisor is
   A. acceptable if you are sick.
   B. acceptable at the end of your shift, even if no other caregiver has arrived to take your place.
   C. known as abandonment.
   D. important to you.

4. If a nursing assistant leaves the side rails down and a helpless patient is seriously injured,
   A. the nursing assistant is guilty of malpractice.
   B. there is no breach of duty.
   C. the nursing assistant is protected under the Good Samaritan Act.
   D. the nursing assistant may be charged with negligence.

5. Putting a patient in a restraining device without a written doctor's order is known as
   A. invasion of privacy.
   B. liability.
   C. false imprisonment.
   D. a prudent practice.

6. A person can give written instructions in advance that life-support systems shall not be used in the event that they ~~are sick.~~
   A. True
   B. False
   Correct Answer: _Near Death_

7. Voluntary acts by which a conscious and mentally competent person gives permission for someone else to do something for him is known as a civil law.
   A. True
   B. False
   Correct Answer: _~~can~~ Informed Concent_

8. A quality shown by coming to work every day on time and doing what is asked at the proper time and in the proper way is known as
   A. good hygiene.
   B. malpractice.
   C. liability.
   D. dependability.
9. When professionals, such as registered nurses, are negligent, they can be charged with
   A. the patient's hospital bill.
   B. an advance directive.
   C. impersonating a Good Samaritan.
   D. malpractice.
10. The document from the American Hospital Association describing the basic rights to which a patient is entitled is known as
   A. the Good Samaritan Act.
   B. the Hospital Bill of Rights.
   C. a living will.
   D. the Patient's Bill of Rights.

COMMUNICATION SKILLS

The following exercises will assist you to apply what you have read in Chapter 3, "Communication Skills." For each exercise, read the objective and use information you have read in Chapter 3 to answer the questions, complete the sentences, or label the diagrams.

EXERCISE 3-1

Objective: To recognize and correctly spell words related to communication skills.

Directions: Unscramble the words in the Word List at the left. Then circle the same words in the Word Search at the right.

Word List

1. BSJUTCEVEI _Subjective_ ✓
2. OJECBVETI _Objective_ ✓
3. YOBD GNAULGAE _Body Language_ ✓
4. EPROTR _Report_ ✓
5. SERBVOE _Observe_ ✓
6. SEDRCBIE _Describe_ ✓
7. VRNOBNALE _Nonverbal_ ✓
8. RITTNWE _Written_ ✓

Word Search

```
N O N V E R B A L L O T D N A
J H I P Q T Z M V E R P Q G D
N T L O X V N G B O E R E H E
M L W A K B U T F V J G C B S
P G D U V D H L I N A H I E C
B R W C W X F T S U P R C M R
S X I E M R O G G P E D O B I
Q B O G X E S N X P B N L I B
F Q H L J X A Q O B S E R V E
M D Q B A L J R C S A D J D C
C L U R Y S T E N U T Q E A O
E S T D E G M N W R I T T E N
H O O Z A I Y J N R B D A F F
I B S O B J E C T I V E K G E
K R L C U Y K X Y V M G Y N O
```

EXERCISE 3-2

Objective: To apply what you have learned about methods of observation.

Directions: Read the following riddles carefully before writing the correct answer on the blank line.

1. If the patient complained about spots and flashes, what area of his body is involved, and what sense would you be interested in observing? *Hint:* It isn't the skin or the sense of touch. __Head + eyes__
2. This could be an important sign of internal bleeding. *Hint:* It resembles something used to brew a morning beverage. __coffee grounds__

3. What would you suspect if the patient you were conversing with yesterday now only nods and smiles at everything you say? *Hint:* You will often find this in the patient's bedside table drawer. __hearing aid__

EXERCISE 3-3

Objective: To recognize the definitions of words related to communication skills that the nursing assistant will use in patient care.

Directions: Place the letter of the correct definition next to the matching word from the Word List.

Word List	Definitions
✓ __D__ 1. tact	A. A familiar phrase used without thinking about what one is saying
✓ __J__ 2. observation	B. Communication through hand movements (gestures), facial expressions, body movements, and touch
✓ __N__ 3. subjective observation	C. The exchange of thoughts, messages, or ideas by speech, signals, gestures, or writing between two or more people
— __O__ 4. subjective reporting	D. Being polite and considerate
✓ __F__ 5. edema	E. When the skin looks blue or gray, especially on the lips, nailbeds, and under the fingernails; in a black patient, it may appear as a darkening of color: this occurs when there is not enough oxygen in the blood.
✓ __C__ 6. communication	F. Abnormal swelling of a part of the body caused by fluid collecting in that area; usually the swelling is in the ankles, legs, hands, or abdomen
✓ __H__ 7. objective observations	G. The ability to put yourself in another's place and to see things as they see them
✓ __B__ 8. body language	H. Signs that can be observed and reported exactly as they are seen
✓ __D__ 9. courtesy	J. Reporting exactly what you observe

___M___ 10. secretions

___E___ 11. cyanosis

___G___ 12. empathy

___I___ 13. objective reporting

___K___ 14. pediatric patient

___L___ 15. feedback

___D___ _A_ 16. cliché

J. Gathering information about the patient by noticing any change

K. Any patient under the age of 16 years

L. Response of the receiver to the sender's message; the response lets the sender know if the message is acknowledged and clearly understood

M. The substances that flow out of or are produced by glandular organs; the process of producing this substance; for example: sweat, bile, lymph, saliva, or urine

N. Symptoms that can be felt and described only by the patient himself, such as pain, nausea, dizziness, ringing in the ears, and headache

O. Giving your opinion about what you have observed; the nursing assistant should never use subjective reporting

P. Doing or saying the right thing at the right time

EXERCISE 3-4

Objective: To demonstrate appropriate responses to changes in the patient's condition.

Directions: Read the situation description and then circle the appropriate response.

1. You have been taking care of Mrs. Jones, 101-A bed, for the last two days. Mrs. Jones has been able to get out of bed and brush her teeth in the bathroom; however, today she says to you, "I will brush my teeth later. I don't feel so good today. I am going to stay in bed. Don't bring me any breakfast." What would you say?
   A. "Stay in bed and later you can get out and brush."
   B. "Are you comfortable? Would you like another blanket? I will be back in half an hour to see how you are feeling." The nursing assistant then goes to the nurse or immediate supervisor to report this change in the patient's condition.
   C. "If you don't brush for one day, it will not hurt you."
   D. "When you give in to feeling sick, you will become very sick."

2. Mr. Murray, the patient in room 209-C bed, had four bowel movements in the last two hours. The last time he wasn't able to wait for the bedpan and soiled the bed. Yesterday, he had one bowel movement the entire day. After you have cleaned the patient and changed his bed, what would you do?
   A. Nothing.
   B. Report this to your nurse or immediate supervisor; this is a definite change in the patient's condition.
   C. Tell the patient he is awful for messing up the bed.
   D. Tell the doctor that the patient has moved his bowels in bed.

3. Mrs. Hernandez, the patient in room 103-A bed, is receiving a blood transfusion that has been running for the past hour. As you are making her bed, you notice that the color of the patient's face is changing. She now has very red cheeks. Mrs. Hernandez cannot speak English and you cannot converse with her. You then notice that Mrs. Hernandez is scratching her arms and legs and seems very agitated. What would you do?

A. Tell the doctor that Mrs. Hernandez is scratching her arms and legs.

B. Tell the patient's visitors to tell her to stop scratching.

C. Use body language so that Mrs. Hernandez will understand and stop scratching.

D. Use the emergency signal to call for help. Report on the intercom to the nurse or immediate supervisor that Mrs. Hernandez seems to be having a reaction to her treatment, and you need help with this patient.

4. A patient complains to you that his "IV hurts." You look at the area on the patient's arm around the needle, and it appears red and swollen. What would you do?

A. Nothing. As a nursing assistant, this is not your job.

B. Tell the patient to mention it to the nurse next time she comes in.

C. Report this immediately to your nurse or immediate supervisor. Although a nursing assistant does not regulate IVs, you still must be observant and report anything unusual.

D. Tell the doctor.

5. Communication is basic to the mutual exchanges of messages that make a connection between the nursing assistant and the patient. What types of things would you do to show good communication skills?

A. Show an interest in what the patient is saying.

B. Speak in a pleasant tone.

C. Use good manners, courtesy, emotional control, sympathy, empathy, and tact.

D. All of the above.

6. Your patient appears to be very irritable. What would you do?

A. Try to calm him down.

B. Try to be an attentive, sympathetic listener.

C. Report this excessive irritability to the nurse or immediate supervisor.

D. Answer the patient in the same irritable manner.

7. Mrs. Smith is a preoperative patient. She is scheduled to go to the operating room in the morning. You notice that when the nurse or immediate supervisor is not around, Mrs. Smith drinks whiskey right from a bottle she keeps in her bedside table. What would you do?

A. Tell the patient to stop drinking.

B. Report this to your nurse or immediate supervisor right away.

C. Tell the patient's visitors that Mrs. Smith is drinking.

D. Tell the doctor that the patient is drinking.

8. Your patient has just been admitted to the health care institution. The doctor ordered oxygen by face mask for this patient. You notice that as soon as the nurse or immediate supervisor leaves the room, the patient takes the mask off. What would you do?

   A. Tell the doctor.

   B. Report this to the nurse or immediate supervisor right away.

   C. Tell another nursing assistant.

   D. Call the pharmacy.

9. Your patient is in the health care institution because of a diabetic condition. The doctor ordered a special therapeutic diet for her. You notice the patient eating a candy bar when she is alone. What would you do?

   A. Let her eat it; she really does not want to get well.

   B. Tell the patient she should not eat the candy without the nurse or immediate supervisor's permission.

   C. Report this incident to your nurse or immediate supervisor, who will tell you what to do.

   D. Ignore the whole thing.

10. Your objective is to report your observations. What would you do in reporting observations of your patient?

   A. Tell the nurse or immediate supervisor what you think is wrong with the patient.

   B. Tell the nurse or immediate supervisor to give the patient some pills.

   C. Tell the nurse or immediate supervisor exactly what you saw, smelled, or felt or what the patient said.

   D. Tell the nurse or immediate supervisor to observe the patient.

11. The nurse or immediate supervisor has given you instructions to report exactly what the patient eats at mealtime and not to give the patient anything between meals. However, during visiting hours, you notice that the patient is eating a hot dog that was brought in by a visitor. What would you do?

   A. Speak to the patient and take the food away immediately.

   B. Call the visitors outside the room and send them home.

   C. Call the doctor and tell him.

   D. Report this to the nurse or immediate supervisor right away.

12. Your patient was fine this morning and was able to get out of bed and walk around his room. However, after lunch, you notice that the patient is lying very quietly in his bed, does not answer when you talk to him, and his face is very red. What would you do?

   A. Shake the patient to wake him every five minutes for one hour.

   B. Call the visitors in to see the patient.

   C. Call the doctor.

   D. Report this to the nurse or immediate supervisor right away; this is a change in the patient's condition.

EXERCISE 3-5

Objective: To demonstrate appropriate communication skills.

Directions: Circle the appropriate response to the following patient situations.

1. You have raised the bedside rails on the bed of a newly admitted woman who is 70 years old. She says, "What are you trying to do, put me in a crib?" The nursing assistant should respond by saying:

    A. "It is the hospital's policy to have the bedside rails up for all patients over the age of 65."

    B. "Does it seem like a crib to you?"

    C. "Don't you want them up?"

    D. "It may seem like a crib to you but it is really because we do not want you to fall. Our beds are high and probably narrower than you are used to."

2. A patient rings his call bell at mealtime. The nursing assistant answers the signal and the patient angrily says, "What's wrong with this place? I have no fork and my coffee is cold!" The nursing assistant should respond by saying:

    A. "I'll do something about it."

    B. "I'll see that you get a fork and hot coffee as soon as I can."

    C. "The dietary department must have a lot of new help."

    D. "Well, that's the way it is around here."

3. A patient signals by ringing the call bell every 15 to 20 minutes. The nursing assistant responds and notices that the patient is making a lot of small requests, such as: "Please raise the window shade"; "Please lower the window shade"; "Please turn on the radio"; "Please turn my pillow." The nursing assistant should respond by:

    A. telling the patient politely not to ring so often.

    B. deliberately delaying in answering the call signal or neglecting to answer it at all.

    C. explaining to the patient that she has other work to do.

    D. reporting to the immediate supervisor, asking what to do, how to handle the situation, and asking the nurse to visit the patient; something is obviously wrong.

4. Mrs. White, a nursing assistant, finished her assignment and is walking down the hall toward the nurses' lounge when another nursing assistant approaches her and says, "Please get Mrs. Smalling in 203-B back to bed for me now. Her doctor is on the nursing unit in another room and wants to examine her. Thank you, Mrs. White, as I have to go and get the dressing cart for the nurse so the doctor can change my patient's bandages." The nursing assistant on her way to the lounge should respond by saying:

    A. "That's not my job, since it is not my patient."

    B. "I will do this right away. By the time you get to Mrs. Smalling's room, she will be in bed."

    C. "I am going to complain to the nurse that you are always asking me to do your work."

    D. "I am tired from my own assignment, and if this hospital wants me to do two jobs, let them pay me two salaries."

5. The nursing assistant has just been told by the nurse that walking to the linen closet five times during one patient's bed bath is bad technique, time-consuming, and not acceptable. One trip should be made, and all the linen needed for one patient must be brought into the room at one time. The nursing assistant should respond by saying:

A. "Thank you for taking the time to teach me. I will try your suggestion now that I understand that what I have been doing is not acceptable. I am sure that my feet will feel better if I do not do so much walking."

B. "How dare you criticize me!"

C. "I went to school to learn how to be a nursing assistant, and you have no right to tell me how to do anything."

D. "You always manage to think of something else I do that you do not like; this is the fourth time this morning that you have told me that I am doing something wrong."

6. Miss Smith, a nursing assistant, is told to go to 201-A bed to give the patient, Mrs. Joseph, a message from her family. Miss Smith has never met this patient, and even though other staff members refer to all of the patients by room and bed number, she does not feel this is right. What would be the right way for Miss Smith to greet the patient?

A. "Are you 201-A bed? Your husband called. . . ."

B. "How do you do, Mrs. Joseph. I am Miss Smith, a nursing assistant. May I check your identification bracelet? Thank you. The nurse asked me to give you this message. . . ."

C. "Hi, your husband called. . . ."

D. "Hi, are you the diabetic patient? Well, I have a message for you. . . ."

EXERCISE 3-6

Objective: To apply what you have learned about good communication techniques.

Directions: Write the word *Do* or *Don't* next to each statement below as appropriate.

1. Don't use a shrill or loud voice, especially if the patient does not speak the same language as you do.

2. Do speak clearly and slowly, especially to hearing-impaired patients.

3. Don't speak in a harsh manner so that the patient will not bother you as often.

4. Don't use medical terms and abbreviations when talking with patients.

5. Don't use age-specific communication styles.

6. Don't let the patient think you are too busy to listen, even if you are.

7. Do respect the patient's cultural preferences.

8. Do show an interest in what the patient is saying.

9. Don't use slang words or clichés.

10. Do speak using a pleasant tone of voice.

EXERCISE 3-7

Objective: To apply what you have learned about communication with patients, families, and your health care team members.

Directions: Circle the letter next to the statement that best completes the sentence or describes the sentence as true or false. If the sentence is false, draw a line through the incorrect part of the sentence and write the correction on the blank line.

1. Both verbal and nonverbal communication involve three important elements:
   A. a criticizer, a moderator, and an evaluator.
   B. a host, an audience, and a sponsor.
   C. a stretcher, a toner, and an exerciser.
   D. a sender, a receiver, and a message.

2. The sender must send a clear meassage.
   A. True
   B. False
   Correct Answer: _____

3. The receiver should ask for clarification if necessary.
   A. True
   B. False
   Correct Answer: _____

4. When working with patients, the message should be unclear, disorganized, and complicated in order to challenge the listening skills of the receiver.
   A. True
   B. False
   Correct Answer: should be clear, organized, _____

5. An example of good body language to use when providing care to a patient is to
   A. pause briefly to ask, "How are you?" and then leave quickly before the reply is completed.
   B. back slowly out of the room as you are talking.
   C. glance out the window often while speaking to the patient about his level of pain.
   D. look directly at the arm the patient is describing as painful.

6. A key to good communication is to be _____ when you listen.
   A. talking
   B. nonjudgmental
   C. ready to reply
   D. opinionated

7. To distract the child when he is unhappy or fearful means to
   A. discipline him for crying.
   B. turn his attention to other things, such as a toy or book.
   C. tell him to be happy.
   D. contact the parents immediately.

8. Being sensitive to times when a patient may not want to talk means
   A. you sing happy songs so he won't feel he has to talk to you.
   B. you convey your support with positive body language instead of carrying on a conversation with him.
   C. you encourage him to "talk things over" with you so he will feel better.
   D. you should be offended that he does not talk to you.

9. Pediatric patients are sometimes grouped according to age because
   A. children of different ages play well together.
   B. children of different ages need different kinds of care.
   C. children age differently.
   D. children do better if grouped.

10. A smile can communicate many positive things to a child.
    A. True
    B. False
    Correct Answer: _____

11. Addressing adults in the manner they prefer, such as "Mrs. Smith" rather than "Grandma," shows that you respect them as people.
    A. True
    B. False
    Correct Answer: _____

12. For pediatric patients, all of the following are true except
    A. Family members need to be with their children.
    B. Most children first learn about the world from their families.
    C. Family members are normally concerned about the child.
    D. The less serious the illness, the less they need their family.

13. If you suspect the child has been abused by the family,
    A. ask them if they have stopped beating the child.
    B. report your suspicions and any objective observations to your immediate supervisor at once.
    C. call 911.
    D. take the child away from them immediately.

14. It is helpful to make visitors feel welcome by pleasant comments about
    A. their appearance.
    B. flowers or gifts they may give you.
    C. flowers or gifts they may bring for the patient.
    D. the new, shorter visiting hours.

15. When visitors bring food for the patient,
    A. you must taste the food before the patient eats it.
    B. ask if you may have some.
    C. tell them it is not allowed.
    D. find out if the nurse or doctor has approved this practice.

16. If your patient is visually impaired, make sure you
    A. have him demonstrate to you that he can use the call light.
    B. leave the call light on the bedside table.
    C. remind him to shut off the light.
    D. All of the above.

17. Communicating with hearing- or speaking-impaired patients is helped by the use of a pad of paper and a pencil to communicate in writing.
    A. True
    B. False
    Correct Answer: _____

18. If your patient speaks a different language or needs sign language, your employer or institution must address that need.
    A. True
    B. False
    Correct Answer: _____

19. A _____ has pictures of the patient's equipment and is a tool to help you communicate with the patient.
    A. story board
    B. outboard
    C. communication board
    D. notice board

20. Incidents, such as a patient fall, should be reported to your immediate supervisor as soon as you
    A. have time to do so after your break.
    B. observe it or it is reported to you.
    C. can after completing your daily assignment.
    D. can after discussing it with the patient's family.

21. As a nursing assistant, you should be aware of the _____ in your institution so that you can follow it when you or others have a complaint that must be resolved by your employer.
    A. grievance procedure
    B. problem roadmap
    C. critical pathway
    D. case management process

PATIENTS, RESIDENTS, AND CLIENTS

The following exercises will assist you to apply what you have read in Chapter 4, "Patients, Residents, and Clients." For each exercise, read the objective and use information you have read in Chapter 4 to answer the questions, complete the sentences, or label the diagrams.

EXERCISE 4-1

Objective: To recognize and correctly spell words related to the care of patients, residents, and clients.

Directions: Unscramble the words in the Word List at the left. Then circle the same words in the Word Search at the right.

Word List

1. TOMCSRUE _____Customer_____
2. RSVEIEC _____Service_____
3. TNMUE SDNEE _____unmet needs_____
4. TLUUCRE _____Culture_____
5. NGLAAUGE _____Language_____
6. IBLEEFS _____Beliefs_____
7. HEBVIAOR _____BEHAVIOR_____
8. TYREISIDV _____Diversity_____

Word Search

R	G	T	P	I	K	C	S	F	D	L	C	M
K	S	I	K	N	O	Z	E	A	G	B	U	Y
Z	V	M	A	B	U	F	X	F	L	E	S	J
C	M	I	L	W	E	X	I	D	G	J	T	K
L	E	S	E	R	V	I	C	E	C	I	O	F
C	Q	D	O	G	L	P	J	A	H	B	M	A
U	N	M	E	T	N	E	E	D	S	Y	E	P
L	A	N	G	U	A	G	E	N	C	T	R	N
T	B	F	H	J	E	C	L	D	T	I	H	D
U	S	B	B	E	L	I	E	F	S	S	C	E
R	I	J	D	F	M	D	L	B	N	R	A	F
E	M	A	O	G	R	B	O	D	G	E	G	D
O	D	Q	H	D	J	A	F	I	J	V	I	B
I	B	E	H	A	V	I	O	R	K	I	H	K
F	K	C	O	H	L	B	R	A	G	D	L	O

EXERCISE 4-2

Objective: To apply what you have learned about patients, residents, and clients.

Directions: Read the following riddles carefully before writing the correct answer on the blank line.

1. What are the thoughts, beliefs, and values of a social group called? *Hint:* An alternative meaning is something that is very active in yogurt. Culture

2. These are people who receive patient care. *Hint:* A salesperson values them. Customers

3. If you are fearful, you may want this on at night when trying to sleep. *Hint:* The opposite of heavy. Light

EXERCISE 4-3

Objective: To recognize the definitions of words related to the care of patients, residents, and clients.

Directions: Place the letter of the correct definition next to the matching word from the word list below.

Word List	Definition
E 1. resident	A. The thoughts, beliefs, and values of a social group
C 2. ethnic diversity	B. A requirement for survival
H 3. service	C. The variety of races, religions, and cultures in the world
B 4. need	D. Care designed to meet the needs of patients, residents, and clients (customers)
G 5. physical crisis management	E. An individual cared for in a nursing home or other long-term/extended care facility
A 6. culture	F. An individual cared for by a home health agency or provider
I 7. client	G. Factors such as attentiveness, quality of food, and cleanliness of environment that affect the care and comfort of the individual receiving health care
F 8. patient	H. Methods for dealing with a dangerous situation involving a patient, resident, or client
D 9. customer focused care	I. An individual admitted to an inpatient or outpatient hospital, physician office, or clinic

EXERCISE 4-4

Objective: To recognize important components of care given to patients, residents, and clients.

Directions: Place the correct letters next to the matching phrase. More than one answer may apply.

> CF = customer focused care goal   SS = sleep stages
> FAS = factors affecting sleep

FAS 1. Keep door closed at night to reduce noise.
CF 2. Information is communicated.
SS 3. Body rests and restores.
FAS 4. Patient may not be comfortable with her roommate, so a change may be needed.
SS 5. Muscles completely relax.
CF 6. Care provided reflects respect for the individual.
FAS 7. Avoid exertion less than two hours prior to sleeping time.
CF 8. Family and friends are involved.
SS 9. Vivid dreaming.
FAS CF 10. The patient is relieved of fear when possible.
FAS 11. Easily aroused.
FAS 12. May be allowed to have own pillow from home.
SS 13. Lower vital signs.
CF 14. Caregivers work together in a planned way.
SS 15. Sound sleep.

EXERCISE 4-5

Objective: To recognize the appropriate response to disruptive behavior.

Directions: Circle the correct response for the disruptive behavior.

1. Patient is angry: A. Remain calm.   B. Frown and shout at them.
2. Patient is stressed: A. Be supportive.   B. Ignore them.
3. Patient has emotional problems: A. Increase stimuli.   B. Focus on safety.

EXERCISE 4-6

Objective: To apply what you have learned about patients, residents, and clients.

Directions: Circle the letter next to the word or statement that best completes the sentence or describes the sentence as true or false. If the sentence is false, draw a line through the incorrect part of the sentence and write the correction on the blank line.

1. Patients, families, and visitors will judge the care given to their loved ones based on all of the following except
   A. personal interactions and attentiveness.
   B. perceived helpfulness of the staff.
   C. employee behavior and quality of the food.
   D. the name of the nursing assistant.

2. Dissatisfied customers may not complain, but they may often return to the same institution.
   A. True
   B. False
   Correct Answer: _they May not Return_

3. Dissatisfied customers will complain to an average of _____ other relatives, friends, or acquaintances.
   A. 4
   B. 7
   C. 200
   D. 20

4. There are seventeen goals of customer focused care.
   A. True
   B. False
   Correct Answer: _____

5. Ethnic diversity is decreasing in the United States.
   A. True
   B. False
   Correct Answer: _increasing_

6. Currently, one in every four Americans is
   A. ethnically deprived.
   B. culturally defined.
   C. Hispanic, Chinese, or Asian.
   D. Hispanic, African American, or Asian.

7. The patients a nursing assistant cares for may have
   A. cultural similarities.
   B. cultural differences.
   C. both cultural similarities and differences.
   D. all of the above.

8. "Different" means the wrong way of doing things.
   A. True
   (B.) False
   Correct Answer: _Doesn't mean it wrong_

9. To be respectful of your patient's cultural differences you should _____ rather than evaluate his behavior.
   A. listen
   B. observe
   C. describe
   D. all of the above

10. _____ are not easily translated into other languages, cultures, or value systems and are usually misunderstood.
    (A.) Directions
    B. Songs
    C. Poems
    D. Jokes

11. Part of the job of the nursing assistant is to try to show the patient that the health care institution is a friendly place and that the major concern is for their
    A. discharge.
    B. well-being.
    (C.) cure.
    D. cultural diversity.

12. It is a good idea to use culturally diverse gestures often when communicating, even if you're not sure what they may mean to the patient.
    (A.) True
    B. False
    Correct Answer: _____

13. If your patient appears upset because of difficulty in communication, you should
    A. explain to him that the care team is friendly.
    B. report this to your immediate supervisor.
    C. speak louder.
    (D.) write the directions on a flash card.

14. Because of cultural differences regarding modesty, it is a good idea to
    A. drape the patient's entire body at all times to be safe.
    (B.) ask your immediate supervisor for suggestions to protect the patient's modesty.
    C. ask the patient to stop being so different.
    D. keep the nursing assistant draped at all times.

15. All patient needs must be met every day by the nursing assistant.
    (A.) True
    B. False
    Correct Answer: _____

16. In Maslow's hierarchy, _____ needs must be met before higher-level needs.
    A. lower-level
    B. middle-level
    C. end-level
    D. beginning-level

17. An example of a lower-level need is
    A. food.
    B. music.
    C. belonging.
    D. leaving.

18. Unmet needs can cause people to show some reaction, such as
    A. anger.
    B. depression.
    C. weakness.
    D. all of the above.

19. Observe the patient's behavior carefully, so that you can report it
    A. subjectively.
    B. continually.
    C. objectively.
    D. quickly.

20. It is during sleep that
    A. work gets done.
    B. time stands still.
    C. tissues heal.
    D. life goes on.

21. Individuals have different _____ clocks.
    A. alarm
    B. body
    C. cultural
    D. biological

22. Whenever possible, plan care to accommodate the individual's sleep preferences.
    A. True
    B. False
    Correct Answer: _____

23. People need to spend enough time in _____ sleep each night to feel rested.
    A. ABC
    B. REM
    C. RAP
    D. EYE

24. The nursing assistant must make _____ a priority when dealing with disruptive patients or families.
    A. safety
    B. humor
    C. speed
    D. sleep

25. Remember that many people want their "say," not their
    A. "pay."
    B. "way."
    C. "day."
    D. "play."

INFECTION CONTROL

The following exercises will assist you to apply what you have read in Chapter 5, "Infection Control." For each exercise, read the objective and use information you have read in Chapter 5 to answer the questions, complete the sentences, or label the diagrams.

EXERCISE 5-1

Objective: To recognize and correctly spell words related to infection control.

Directions: Unscramble the words in the Word List at the left. Then circle the same words in the Word Search at the right.

Word List

1. GNESHOPTA — _Pathogens_
2. IHSO — _____
3. SRECOU — _Source_
4. RTSNAMSISION — _Transmission_
5. IONTLASIO — _Isolation_
6. DHWNASHAGNI — _Handwashing_
7. TCIFRNIO — _Friction_
8. TITPHEAIS — _Hepatitis_

Word Search

P	A	T	H	O	G	E	N	S	S	A	B	L	I	E	O
A	L	V	O	P	Y	Z	L	Q	C	K	M	K	Q	Z	A
E	N	V	S	O	U	R	C	E	F	G	H	Z	H	F	D
X	S	C	T	R	A	N	S	M	I	S	S	I	O	N	L
K	I	D	K	V	L	A	X	E	T	M	T	E	V	X	D
O	G	S	E	B	T	L	B	E	S	F	O	W	B	C	B
C	I	R	O	I	V	G	J	I	H	R	J	S	S	E	Y
A	K	M	E	L	H	G	L	S	B	I	A	J	I	G	Z
D	W	O	W	D	A	A	P	N	E	C	H	S	T	P	O
H	S	J	T	G	N	T	M	S	Z	T	N	I	I	C	H
D	F	X	B	S	D	K	I	B	E	I	E	K	T	M	B
M	B	K	M	Q	W	I	S	Q	C	O	H	H	A	A	L
R	L	F	P	Z	A	N	P	G	N	N	D	F	P	L	E
A	I	L	C	R	S	L	D	H	V	T	T	Y	E	F	N
N	W	P	A	N	H	E	Y	V	L	D	N	A	H	I	K
H	N	W	H	S	I	S	G	M	X	S	F	R	P	E	G
J	C	F	T	S	N	H	C	A	K	J	C	M	B	D	E
F	O	D	K	J	G	N	T	D	P	S	G	H	Z	A	C
X	G	K	I	J	T	F	B	E	G	M	F	E	I	D	A

EXERCISE 5-2

Objective: To apply what you have learned about infection control.

Directions: Read the following riddles carefully before writing the correct answer on the blank line.

1. Put me on your skin or an object and I will kill many microorganisms as I disappear. *Hint:* Sometimes you will call me by a name that sounds like a woman's name but is spelled differently. *Ethyl alchol*
2. Without this process we would never be a host. *Hint:* An automobile has one of these. *Transmission*
3. This word means "free of disease-producing organisms." *Hint:* The word would mean quite the opposite if you dropped the first letter. *Aseptic*

EXERCISE 5-3

Objective: To recognize the definitions of words related to infection control.

Directions: Place the letter of the correct definition next to the matching word from the Word List.

Word List		Definitions
N 1. virus		A. Germ free, without disease-producing organisms
H 2. asepsis		B. Device used to achieve sterility of an item through heat, pressure, and steam
G 3. infection		C. Unicellular microorganism
J 4. nosocomial infection		D. The process of destroying as many harmful organisms as possible
C 5. bacteria		E. The process of rubbing two surfaces together, such as skin
E 6. friction		F. Blood-borne disease that affects the liver and is easily transmitted within the health care setting following parenteral exposure
B 7. autoclave		G. Due to a pathogen producing a reaction which may cause soreness, tenderness, redness, and/or pus, fever, change in drainage, and so on
M *D* 8. sterilization		H. The absence of microorganisms
F 9. hepatitis B		I. A living thing that is so small it cannot be seen with the naked eye but only through a microscope
D *M* 10. disinfection		J. Hospital acquired infection
L 11. spores		K. Disease producing microorganism
A 12. aseptic		L. Bacteria that have formed hard shells around themselves as a defense

_K_ 13. pathogen

_I_ 14. microorganism

_M._ The process of killing all microorganisms, including spores

_N._ A type of microorganism that is much
smaller than bacteria and can survive
only in other living cells

EXERCISE 5-4

Objective: To apply what you have learned about disinfection and steril-
ization.

Directions: Look at Figure 5-1; then circle the letter of the correct
answer for each question.

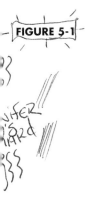

FIGURE 5-1

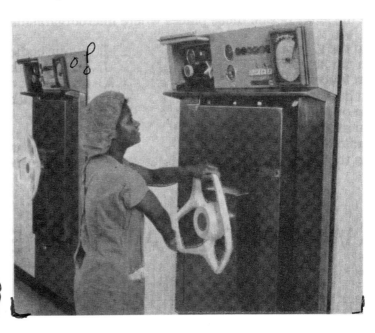

1. The machine in Figure 5-1 is called a/an
   A. sterilizer.
   B. autoclave.
   C. pasteurizer.
   D. wheelchair.
   E. suction machine.

2. The autoclave sterilizes or completely destroys microorganisms by com-
bining
   A. soap with hot water under pressure.
   B. acid with steam.
   C. ammonia with steam under pressure.
   D. heat with steam under pressure.
   E. water and bleach under pressure.

3. Autoclaves are used to kill
   A. bad germs only.
   B. all bacteria and viruses, including spores.
   C. parasites.
   D. time.
4. When an object is free of all _____, it is sterile.
   A. grease
   B. worry
   C. wrinkles
   D. microorganisms

EXERCISE 5-5

Objective: To apply what you have learned about the use of patient care precautions and barrier devices, such as disposable gloves and a mask.

Directions: In Figure 5-2, label the steps in the order that you would perform them.

FIGURE 5-2

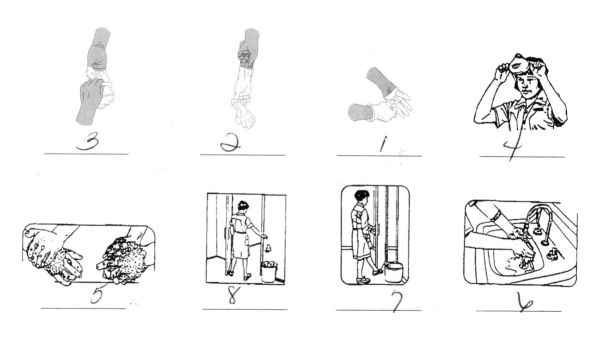

EXERCISE 5-6

Objective: To apply what you have learned about microorganisms and protective barriers.

Directions: Choose the correct method of mask use by putting a circle around either letter A or letter B in Figure 5-3.

FIGURE 5-3

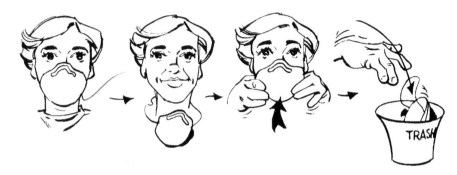

A:

To save money, wear the mask around your neck, and only put it on when you need it during the workday.

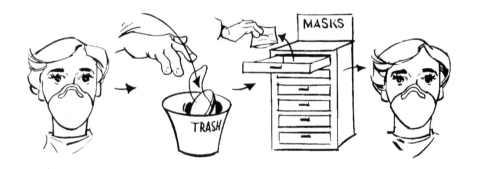

B:

Use each mask only once. Dispose of it when the procedure is complete, and get a clean mask the next time you need one.

EXERCISE 5-7

Objective: To apply what you have learned about infection control.

Directions: Circle the letter next to the word or sentence that best completes the sentence or describes the sentence as true or false. If the sentence is false, draw a line through the incorrect part of the sentence and write the correction on the blank line.

1. The source of microorganisms
   A. can only be the patient and the health care worker.
   B. is never really known.
   C. can be anyone, including objects in the environment.
   D. is a susceptible host only.

2. Standard Precautions are designed to provide safety to
   A. health care workers.
   B. patients.
   C. both A and B.
   D. nursing assistants who are in training.

3. To prevent or control the transmission of diseases, you
   A. must study very hard.
   B. must understand how a disease is spread.
   C. must protect yourself and your patient.
   D. both B and C.

4. Your ability to resist infections depends on your individual
   A. personality.
   B. income.
   C. age.
   D. health status and exposure to a pathogen.

5. To be reinfected means you or your patient have become infected a second time by the same microorganism.
   A. True
   B. False
   Correct Answer: _____

6. Cross infection means becoming infected by a new microorganism from another patient or a health care worker.
   A. True
   B. False
   Correct Answer: _____

7. Standard Precautions apply to
   A. blood, all body fluids, nonintact skin, and mucous membranes.
   B. saliva, semen, and blood.
   C. care of the burned patient.
   D. all of the above.

8. You will not wear gloves if your patient is on Droplet Precautions.
    A. True
    B. False
    Correct Answer: _Wear them_

9. Cleanliness is important, so be sure that your fingernails are
    A. kept short and are cleaned frequently.
    B. colorful and attractive at all times.
    C. kept long to facilitate opening packages.
    D. extended 1/2 inch beyond the ends of your fingers.

10. You have never had chicken pox and you discover your patient is infected with this disease. What do you do?
    A. Hold your breath while caring for this patient.
    B. Wear gloves and a mask to prevent infection in the patient.
    C. You are over 21 and so cannot develop this disease.
    D. You speak to your immediate supervisor about taking a different patient assignment.

11. The key to good handwashing is
    A. hot water.
    B. friction and hand cream to protect against chapping.
    C. bar soap instead of dispensed soap.
    D. adequate soap, lots of tepid water, and friction.

12. During handwashing, if your hands touched the inside of the sink you would
    A. start over.
    B. rinse 30 seconds longer, and use paper towels to wipe the sink.
    C. use adequate paper towels and friction.
    D. ignore it because you have soap on your hands to kill the germs.

13. Gloves provide a complete barrier to contamination.
    A. True
    B. False
    Correct Answer: _Not a complete barrier_

14. _____ is a good technique to use during handwashing.
    A. Transmission
    B. Interlacing
    C. both A and B
    D. Log-rolling

15. Hands must be washed after removing gloves.
    A. True
    B. False
    Correct Answer: _____

COMPETENCY CHECKLIST 5-1: INFECTION CONTROL

ACTIVITY	S	U	COMMENTS
1. Student correctly demonstrates proper handwashing procedure:			
A. Application of soap and water			
B. Use of friction			
C. Use of paper towel to shut off faucets			
2. Student correctly demonstrates proper gloving procedure:			
A. Application of non-sterile disposable gloves			
B. Removal of non-sterile disposable gloves			
C. Application of sterile disposable gloves			
D. Removal of sterile disposable gloves			
3. Student correctly demonstrates proper gowning procedure:			
A. Application of gown			
B. Removal of gown			
4. Student correctly demonstates proper procedure to clean non-critical items:			
A. Not visibly soiled			
B. Visibly soiled			

SAFETY

The following exercises will assist you to apply what you read in Chapter 6, "Safety." For each exercise, read the objective and use information you have read in Chapter 6 to answer the questions, complete the sentences, or label the diagrams.

EXERCISE 6-1

Objective: To recognize and correctly spell words related to safety.

Directions: Unscramble the words in the Word List on the left. Then circle the same words in the Word Search at the right.

Word List

1. YTEFAS _____ Safty ✓
2. STANISTRER _____ Restraints ✓
3. ROAB _____ OBRA ✓
4. RFEI _____ Fire ✓
5. YXENOG _____ Oxygen ✓
6. TNEPVER _____ Prevent ✓
7. SKEABR _____ Brakes ✓
8. ZOARSR _____ Razors

Word Search

A	N	O	R	C	A	D	P	E	J	M	K	K	F	A	H	C
K	S	Q	U	A	Z	L	J	L	G	Q	F	A	L	E	C	D
R	M	V	E	Q	R	F	B	X	H	O	L	J	S	M	F	Z
J	V	S	A	F	E	T	Y	D	F	I	T	D	A	H	I	E
Z	A	F	G	H	S	F	M	I	N	B	J	C	R	O	B	D
P	B	F	C	D	T	J	B	K	A	H	Z	T	V	A	H	G
D	C	I	J	N	R	C	E	N	D	P	E	N	U	X	J	H
X	I	O	B	R	A	H	D	B	R	A	K	E	S	I	G	H
J	K	X	L	F	I	R	E	I	A	D	A	V	M	H	D	B
K	P	Y	R	H	N	F	A	C	Z	F	V	E	J	A	H	K
L	S	G	L	I	T	S	P	J	O	H	S	R	A	Z	L	I
O	M	E	V	C	S	A	I	T	R	L	N	P	P	R	S	D
H	T	N	H	J	G	J	K	S	S	H	L	D	J	V	D	G
M	V	G	Z	A	M	V	O	G	X	I	M	G	F	A	N	A
B	O	D	I	Q	R	A	K	Y	P	K	C	O	Q	H	O	D

EXERCISE 6-2

Objective: To recognize safety issues and immediate actions to be taken.

Directions: Place the correct letters that would apply to the situation next to the matching phrase, then circle the correct response you should take immediately. More than one set of letters can be selected for each situation.

OS = oxygen safety   RS = restraint safety   CS = child safety
FS = fire safety   AS = ambulation safety   PS = patient safety

1. Your patient has nasal oxygen on at 3 liters and there is a NO SMOKING—OXYGEN IN USE sign on the wall above his bed. His wife is preparing to light a candle at the bedside and say a prayer for his recovery. **LETTERS:** _PS/FS/ AS OS_ **What would you do?**
   A. You grab the fire extinguisher and **P**ull the pin, **A**im low, **S**queeze the handle, and **S**weep from side to side, aiming at the base of the candle.
   B. You put out the candle and explain to her that open flames are dangerous when oxygen is running. You offer to show her where the chapel is located.
   C. You turn off the oxygen for 20 minutes until she is done praying.
   D. You ignore the situation because such a small flame is harmless.

2. You are ready to leave for the day and stop in to say good-bye to your patient. She tells you that the floor in the bathroom is wet. You realize that the housekeeping staff has gone home for the day. **LETTERS:** _AS/ PS_ **What would you do?**
   A. You clean up the floor immediately, or get someone else to do it.
   B. You leave immediately, because you must take your sick child to the doctor.
   C. You provide the patient with a call light and instruct her to ask someone on the new shift to do it because you are leaving.
   D. You tell the patient to stay out of the bathroom until someone else comes to clean it up.

3. You are coming on your new shift and notice that one of your patients is wearing a chest restraint that is on backwards. The patient is sleeping at this time. **LETTERS:** _PS /RS_ **What would you do?**
   A. Let him sleep for now.
   B. Make a note to change the restraint later on when you have more time.
   C. Leave a call light within reach.
   D. Check with your immediate supervisor to determine if help is needed when changing the restraint, based on the patient's condition and reason for wearing the restraint. You change the restraint immediately.

4. You notice that your patient, a 7-year-old, is picking at the IV site on his arm. **LETTERS:** _CS_ **What would you do?**
   A. You restrain him immediately.
   B. You report this to your immediate supervisor.
   C. You sit with the child, give him some toys to play with, and report this to your immediate supervisor later that day.
   D. You report this to your supervisor immediately. You stop by often to sit with him, give him some toys, and explain how important it is to not disturb the IV.

5. When getting a patient up to sit at the bedside in a reclining chair, you notice the chair's wheel brakes do not work well. This causes the chair to slide backward about 6 inches across the floor as the patient sits down. The patient is not injured. **LETTERS:** _⟋_ S _____ **What would you do?**

   A. Make out a work repair form and send it to the proper person.

   B. Notify your immediate supervisor, and tell your coworkers to be careful.

   C. Get another chair for your patient. Get help transferring him to the new chair, and remove the broken chair from the patient care area after labeling it "broken." Report this to your immediate supervisor.

   D. Make sure the chair is always up against the wall in the future when you transfer the patient to it, so that he will not be injured when it moves.

6. As you prepare to take Mr. O'Shea for a walk, you notice that the walker he brought from home to use in the hospital has two rubber tips missing from the feet. **LETTERS:** _⟋_ S _____ **What would you do?**

   A. Make a note to have the medical equipment staff take a look at it next time they are in.

   B. Obtain another walker that is the same size and that has all four rubber tips in place before you ambulate him.

   C. Tell his wife to buy some new tips for the walker.

   D. Let him use it this time because he is too impatient to wait for his walk, and you don't want him to complain to the immediate supervisor about you.

EXERCISE 6-3

Objective: To apply what you have learned about safety.

Directions: Circle the letter next to the word or statement that best completes the sentence or describes the sentence as true or false. If the sentence is false, draw a line through the incorrect part of the sentence and write the correction on the blank line.

1. **RACE** stands for

   A. **R**un **A**way and **C**all **E**MS.

   B. **R**emove yourself **A**nd **C**all "Exit!"

   C. **R**un **A**nd **C**orrect the **E**mergency.

   D. **R**emove the patient; **A**ctivate the alarm; **C**ontain the fire; **E**xtinguish the fire if safe to do so.

2. It takes three things to have a fire: heat, fuel, and wind.

   A. True

   B. False

   Correct Answer: _____ Oxygen _____

3. It is important to change the evacuation plan of your facility.

   A. True

   B. False

   Correct Answer: _____ Keep the same _____

4. The Omnibus Reconciliation Act (OBRA) calls any device a restraint that keeps a patient from moving freely or keeps the patient from reaching parts of his body.
   A. True
   B. False
   Correct Answer: _____

5. When the patient is utilizing nasal oxygen, the areas where skin irritation may occur are
   A. any area where the plastic cannula may touch.
   B. only behind the ears.
   C. the nostrils and the eyelids.
   D. behind the neck and the forehead.

6. _____ is the number one cause of fires in health care institutions.
   A. A sleepy patient
   B. A broken electrical cord
   C. Too much oxygen
   D. Smoking

7. A fire extinguisher may be labeled
   A. A for all, B for wood, C for combustion.
   B. only A for paper fires and B for electrical fires.
   C. ABC for "all burning clothing."
   D. ABC for use on any type of fire.

8. Always place used disposable razors
   A. in a red waste basket.
   B. in approved containers.
   C. in recycling bins.
   D. where they can be quickly found for reuse later.

9. Room cleaning supplies should
   A. be left at the bedside at all times.
   B. be labeled and dated before leaving at the bedside.
   C. be stored away from the patient care area.
   D. be kept in the patient's bathroom.

10. Electrical equipment must never come in contact with
    A. heat, fuel, or oxygen.
    B. patients.
    C. the nursing assistant.
    D. water.

COMPETENCY CHECKLIST 6: SAFETY

COMPETENCY CHECKLIST 6: SAFETY

ACTIVITY	S	U	COMMENTS
1. Student will demonstrate the correct method for applying a waist restraint.			
2. Student will demonstrate the correct method for applying a vest restraint.			

IMPORTANT CRITERIA

1. The nurse or therapist will decide what type of restraint is to be used.			
2. Never tie or secure a restraint to any movable part of a bed or chair.			
3. The patient must be checked at least every 30 minutes while restrained, or more often according to the institution's policy.			
4. Carefully check pressure points for reddness or irritation of the skin.			
5. The patient must be released to offer food and liquids, toilet, exercise, and to reposition him.			

BODY MECHANICS: POSITIONING, MOVING, AND TRANSPORTING PATIENTS

The following exercises will assist you to apply what you have read in Chapter 7, "Body Mechanics: Positioning, Moving, and Transporting Patients." For each exercise, read the objective and use information you have read in Chapter 7 to answer the questions, complete the sentences, or label the diagrams.

EXERCISE 7-1

Objective: To recognize and correctly spell words related to body mechanics utilized while positioning, moving, and transporting a patient.

Directions: Unscramble the words in the Word List at the left. Then circle the same words in the Word Search at the right.

Word List

1. ICMHENACS _Mechanics_
2. YOBD _Body_
3. GEIUAFT _Fatigue_
4. JYNUIR _injury_
5. TNIGFLI _Lifting_
6. PLHEESSL _Helpless_
7. RNATSPTOR _Transport_
8. LALF _Fall_

Word Search

M	E	A	B	C	D	O	X	F	J	A	K	L	M
D	E	F	I	J	O	K	B	K	Q	Y	D	I	H
W	D	C	S	I	W	A	J	R	Z	B	E	F	V
T	N	K	H	E	L	P	L	E	S	S	G	T	I
F	A	N	F	A	T	I	G	U	E	R	A	I	L
B	L	P	K	M	N	X	Q	A	J	Z	C	N	U
W	V	A	C	L	E	I	N	J	U	R	Y	G	Y
H	P	M	L	E	X	V	C	F	D	W	D	B	L
Z	F	S	C	Z	F	W	U	S	L	A	V	L	H
X	Q	R	T	P	B	O	D	Y	X	E	A	G	Y
T	R	A	N	S	P	O	R	T	B	F	C	E	Z

EXERCISE 7-2

Objective: To apply what you have learned about using good body mechanics to position, move, and transport patients.

Directions: Read the following riddles carefully before writing the correct answer on the blank line.

1. These two words refer to use of the proper techniques for standing and moving one's body. What are they? *Hint:* If your car was damaged in a collision, you would ask these skilled workers to fix it. Mechan Machines

2. This term can refer to the way a patient walks, or it can describe a device used to support the patient while walking. What is it? *Hint:* It sounds like part of a fence. Gaile Belto

EXERCISE 7-3

Objective: To recognize the definitions of words used in applying good body mechanics to the positioning, moving, and transporting of patients.

Directions: Complete the sentences with the words from the Word List below.

Word List

Trendelenburg's	dorsal recumbent	body mechanics	Fowler's	drape
body alignment	nonambulatory	side-lying	lithotomy	Sims's
knee-chest	supine	bedridden	draping	prone

1. Nonambulatory means not able to walk.
2. Body Alignment refers to the arrangement of the body in a straight line and the placing of portions of the body in correct anatomical position.
3. Bedbound or Bedridden means the patient is unable to get out of bed.
4. Body Mechanics are special ways of standing and moving one's body to make the best use of strength and avoid fatigue.
5. The patient is in Fowlers position when the head of the bed is at a 45°–90° angle.
6. Covering the patient or parts of the patient's body with a sheet, blanket, or other material is called draping the patient.
7. The patient is in lithotomy position when he lies on his back with his legs spread apart and knees bent.
8. When the patient is lying down on his back he is in the dorsal recumbent position.
9. In the Supine position the patient is lying on his back.
10. In the Side lying position the patient is lying on his side.
11. The patient is in Trendelenburg position when the bed or operating table is tilted so that the patient's head is about a foot below the level of his knees.
12. When the patient is lying on his left side with his right knee and thigh drawn up, he is in Sims position. enema
13. A drape is a covering used to provide privacy during an examination or operation.

14. In the _Knee chest_ position the patient assumes a bent posture with the knees and chest touching the examination table or bed.

15. In the _prone_ position the patient is lying on his stomach.

EXERCISE 7-4

Objective: To demonstrate an understanding of correct body mechanics to use when lifting and/or changing position.

Directions: Circle the letters of the pictures in Figure 7-1 that illustrate correct body mechanics.

FIGURE 7-1

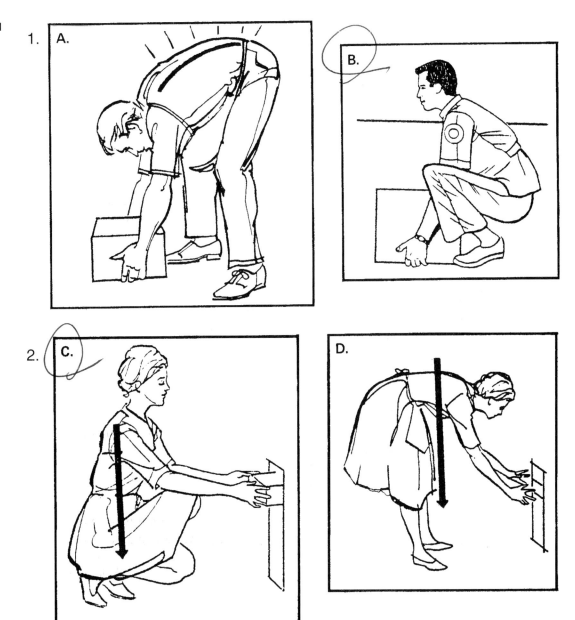

3.

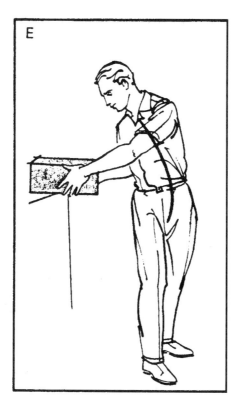
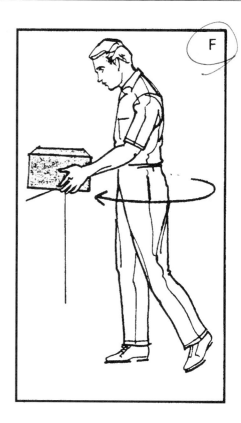

EXERCISE 7-5

Objective: To recognize methods of moving a patient using proper body mechanics.

Directions: Label the pictures in Figure 7-2 with the correct letter from the list that describes the type of moving procedure shown.

List

A. Turning a patient on his side away from you
B. Moving the mattress to the head of the bed with the patient's help
C. Moving a helpless patient to one side of the bed on his back
D. Moving the nonambulatory patient up in bed
E. Turning a patient on his side toward you
F. Moving a patient up in bed with his help

FIGURE 7-2

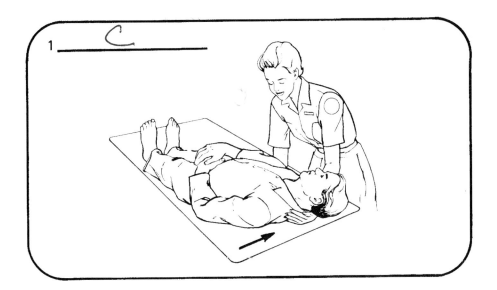

1 _____ C _____

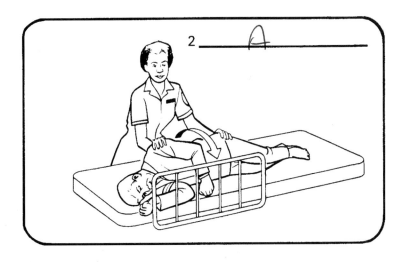

2 _____ A _____

3 _____ B

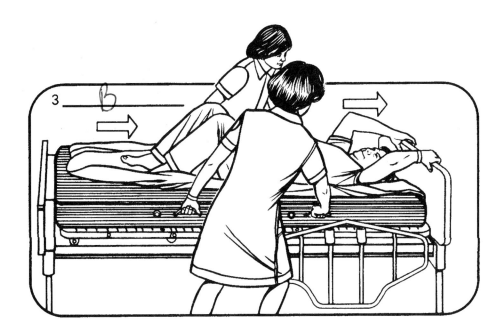

4 _____ D

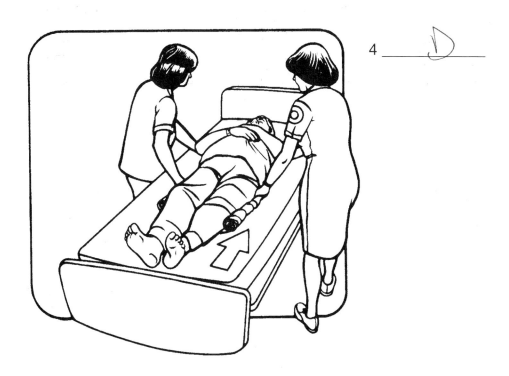

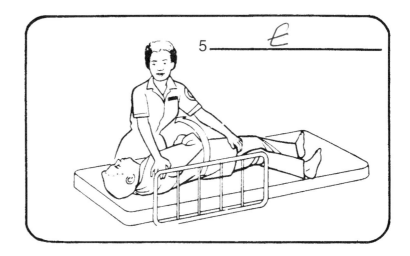

5 _____ E _____

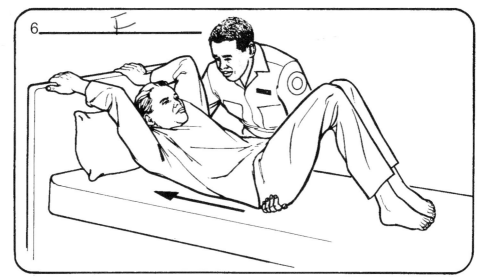

6 _____ F _____

EXERCISE 7-6

Objective: To recognize the proper methods of draping and positioning the patient.

Directions: Label the pictures in Figure 7-3 with the letter from the list that describes the correct method of draping and positioning the patient.

List

A. Horizontal recumbent position
B. Side-lying position
C. Dorsal recumbent position
D. Trendelenburg's position
E. Prone position
F. Reverse Trendelenburg's position

G. Dorsal lithotomy position
H. Fowler's position at 45°
I. Left Sims's position
J. Knee-chest position
K. Left lateral position

FIGURE 7-3

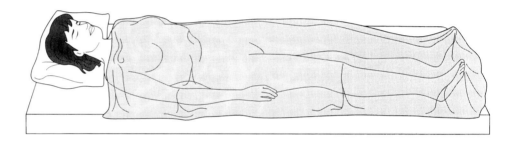

1 ___A___

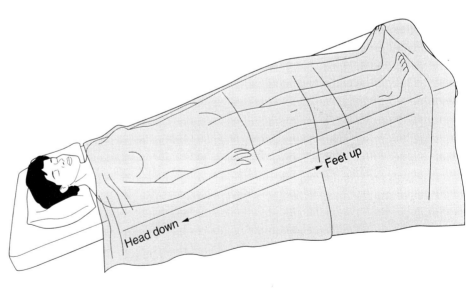

Feet up

Head down

2. ___D___

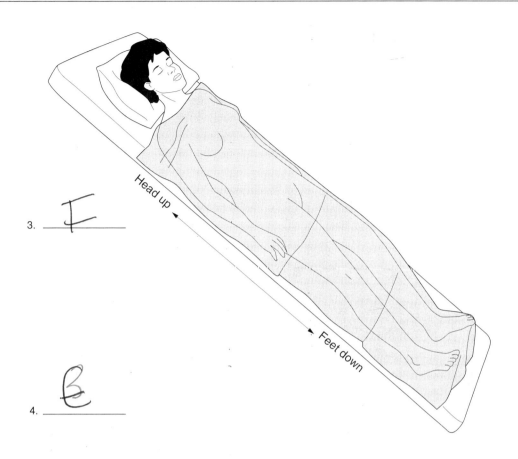

Head up

Feet down

3. _____

4. _____

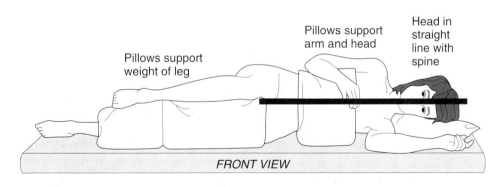

Pillows support
weight of leg

Pillows support
arm and head

Head in
straight
line with
spine

FRONT VIEW

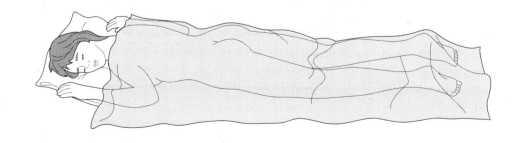

5. _____

6. _____

7. _____

8. _____

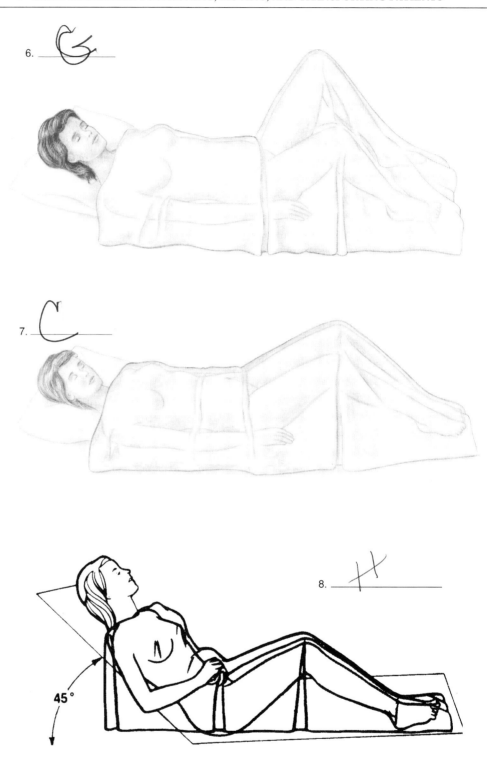

45°

9. _____

10. _____

11. _____

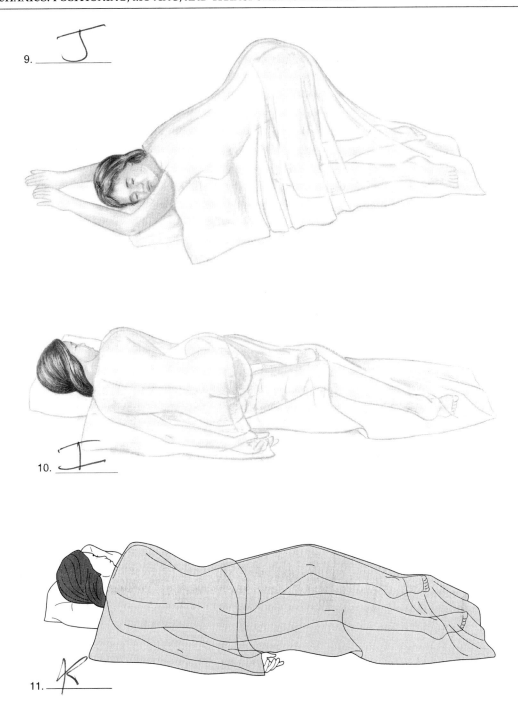

EXERCISE 7-7

Objective: To apply what you have learned about using good body mechanics to position, move, and transport patients.

Directions: Circle the letter next to the statement that best completes the sentence.

1. The term *body mechanics* refers to
   A. the correct positioning of the patient's body.
   B. the bones and joints.
   C. special ways of standing and moving one's body.
   D. artificial arms or legs.
   E. rolling the patient like a log.

2. The purpose of good body mechanics is
   A. to rest comfortably in a hospital bed.
   B. to make the best use of strength and avoid fatigue.
   C. to feel good while losing weight.
   D. to avoid friction and irritation to the patient's skin.
   E. to become stronger and more agile.

3. When an action requires physical effort, you should
   A. get close to the load that is being lifted.
   B. use good posture.
   C. try to use as many muscles or groups of muscles as possible.
   D. ask a friend to do it.
   E. A, B, and C.

4. When lifting an object you should
   A. keep your feet slightly more than hip width apart.
   B. avoid twisting your arms.
   C. squat close to the load.
   D. maintain the natural curves in your back.
   E. all of the above.

5. When you have to move a heavy object
   A. it is better to push it than to lift it.
   B. it is better to pull it than to lift it.
   C. it is better to roll it than to carry it.
   D. it is best to get help from another nursing assistant.
   E. all of the above.

6. The correct positioning of a patient's body is referred to as
   A. body mechanics.
   B. body alignment.
   C. body position.
   D. special patient care treatments.
   E. body arrangement.

EXERCISE 7-8

Objective: To apply what you have learned about lifting and moving patients.

Directions: Fill in the blank spaces with the words from the Word List below.

Word List

friction	position	slide
draw sheet	irritation	roll
folded	bed	grip
under		

A pull sheet can help you move the patient in ___Bed___ more easily. A regular sheet ___folded___ over many times and placed ___under___ the patient can be used as a pull sheet. The cotton ___draw sheet___ can also be used as a pull sheet. When moving the patient, ___roll___ the pull sheet up tightly on each side next to the patient's body. ___Grip___ the rolled portion to ___slide___ the patient into the desired ___position.___ Use of the pull sheet avoids ___friction___ and ___irritation___ to the patient's skin that touches the bedding.

EXERCISE 7-9

Objective: To apply what you have learned about using good body mechanics to position, move, and transport patients.

Directions: Circle the letter next to the statement that best completes the sentence or describes the sentence as true or false. If the sentence is false, draw a line through the incorrect part of the sentence and write the correction on the blank line.

1. When using a gait belt you should position yourself
   A. about 12 inches from the patient.
   B. in front of the patient's stronger side.
   C. in the dorsal recumbent position.
   D. slightly behind the weaker side of the patient.
2. A stretcher should be pushed with the patient's ~~head~~ moving first.
   A. True
   B. False
   Correct Answer: _____feet first_____
3. If a patient begins to fall when you are ambulating him,
   A. bend your back and lower yourself to the floor.
   B. quickly drop to the floor to cushion the patient's fall with your body.
   C. bend your knees and flex your arms.
   D. bend your knees and lower your body to the floor with the patient.

4. When moving a patient in a wheelchair down a steep ramp, you should push the chair down frontwards.
   A. True
   B. False
   Correct Answer: _____ *Backwards* _____

5. When the patient is getting in or out of a _____, both wheels must be locked.
   A. shower
   B. elevator
   C. wheelchair
   D. rocking chair

6. Many conditions and injuries make it dangerous for a patient to be in certain positions.
   A. True
   B. False
   Correct Answer: _____

7. All members of the nursing team are required to know the prescribed position the patient should be in
   A. as ordered by the doctor.
   B. as requested by the family.
   C. as preferred by the patient.
   D. within 2 hours of starting their shift.

8. Before moving the patient, all _____ must be placed where they won't be pulled.
   A. visitors
   B. sheets
   C. tubing (such as catheters and IVs)
   D. pillows

9. A general rule when moving patients is to
   A. drop the arms and legs over the edge of the stretcher.
   B. pull with a quick, jerky movement.
   C. remove all catheters and other tubing.
   D. give the most support to the heaviest parts of the body.

10. Before moving any patient you must
    A. always check the identification bracelet.
    B. rest by taking a break.
    C. notify your immediate supervisor.
    D. be fitted for a gait belt.

COMPETENCY CHECKLIST 7-1: BODY MECHANICS

ACTIVITY	S	U	COMMENTS
1. Student will correctly demonstrate the proper method to move and lift patients:			
A. Moving the helpless patient			
B. Moving a patient up in bed with his help			
C. Moving the mattress to the head of the bed with the patient's help			
D. Moving the helpless patient to one side of the bed on his back			
E. Log rolling the patient			
F. Turning a patient onto his side toward you			
G. Turning a patient onto his side away from you			
H. Repositioning a patient in a chair or wheelchair			
I. Moving the nonambulatory patient into a wheelchair or arm chair from the bed			
J. Helping a nonambulatory patient back into bed from a wheelchair or arm chair			
K. Helping a patient who can stand and is ambulatory back into bed from a chair or a wheelchair			
L. Using a portable mechanical patient lift to move the helpless patient			
M. Moving a patient from the bed to a stretcher			
2. Student will demonstrate the correct method of ambulating a patient:			
A. Using a gait belt			
B. Using a cane, walker, or crutches			
3. Student will demonstrate the correct method of assisting a falling patient.			

ADMITTING, TRANSFERRING, AND DISCHARGING A PATIENT

The following exercises will assist you to apply what you have read in Chapter 8, "Admitting, Transferring, and Discharging a Patient." For each example, read the objective and use information you have read in Chapter 8 to answer the questions, complete the sentences, or label the diagrams.

EXERCISE 8-1

Objective: To recognize the definitions of words related to admitting, transferring, and discharging a patient.

Directions: Place the letter of the correct definition next to the matching word from the Word List.

Word List	Definitions
____ 1. implementing	A. Determining whether a plan (such as the patient care plan) has been effective
____ 2. transfer	B. Gathering facts to identify needs and problems
____ 3. sociocultural	C. The official procedure for helping patients to leave the health care institution, including teaching them how to care for themselves at home
____ 4. physiological	D. Referring to an individual's personal response to inspirational forces.
____ 5. discharge	E. Deciding what to do and how to do it
____ 6. admission	F. A written plan stating the nursing diagnosis, the patient goals or expected outcomes, and the nursing orders, interventions, or actions to be taken
____ 7. spiritual	G. The administrative process that covers the period from the time the patient enters the institution door to the time the patient is settled
____ 8. psychological	H. Carrying out or accomplishing a given plan
____ 9. assessing	I. Moving a hospital patient from one room, unit, or facility to another

____10. holistic

J. Referring to a person's biological response to alterations in the body's structures and functions

____11. patient plan of care

K. The period of recovery after illness or surgery

____12. planning

L. Referring to a person's interpersonal responses to socialization practices in the family and community

____13. evaluating

M. An approach that reflects the four dimensions of a "whole" person: physiological, psychological, sociocultural, and spiritual

____14. convalescence

N. Referring to a person's cognitive and emotional responses to the self and the surrounding environment

EXERCISE 8-2

Objective: To apply what you have learned about admitting, transferring, and discharging a patient.

Directions: Read the following riddles carefully before writing the correct answer on the blank line.

1. All nursing care plans have these to achieve. What are they? *Hint:* In hockey you keep score by counting these. _____
2. This word describes the nursing care plan. What is it? *Hint:* A carpenter has more than one of these in his box. _____
3. These are used to weigh a patient. What are they? *Hint:* Most fish have these. _____

EXERCISE 8-3

Objective: To apply what you have learned about admitting, transferring, and discharging a patient.

Directions: Circle the letter next to the word or statement that best completes the sentence or describes the sentence as true or false. If the sentence is false, draw a line through the incorrect part of the sentence and write the correction on the blank line.

1. At the time of admission, the nursing assistant is very important to the patient because
    A. the patient may be frightened and uncomfortable.
    B. the patient may be in pain.
    C. the patient may be seriously ill.
    D. all of the above.

2. The nursing assistant, by being _____ and _____, will make the patient's admission process easier.
   A. irate, hasty
   B. slow, disorganized
   C. confused, sleepy
   D. pleasant, courteous

3. It is not a good idea to introduce yourself to a patient being admitted even if he is in a lot of pain.
   A. True
   B. False
   Correct Answer: _____

4. The nursing assistant should address the adult patient
   A. with his first name to be informal and friendly.
   B. with his initials only.
   C. as grandma or grandpa to make them feel part of the health care family.
   D. As Mr., Miss, or Ms. and the patient's last name.

5. When admitting a patient, you should keep in mind
   A. the reason for her admission.
   B. the remaining work to be done with other patients.
   C. the tasks the nurse has asked you to do for this patient.
   D. A and C.

6. The nursing assistant is a representative of his institution.
   A. True
   B. False
   Correct Answer: _____

7. An important tool for 24-hour communication for the health care team is the
   A. care strategy log.
   B. physician's log.
   C. nursing care plan.
   D. Internet.

8. The nursing care plan helps the team deliver
   A. the mail.
   B. continuous and consistent care.
   C. floral bouquets.
   D. uncoordinated care.

9. The registered nurse _____ the care plan on admission.
   A. finishes
   B. begins
   C. rejects
   D. approves

10. The registered nurse will identify patient problems and nursing diagnoses.
    A. True
    B. False
    Correct Answer: _____

11. The registered nurse reevaluates the plan of care each day to reflect
    A. the sun.
    B. the changing needs of the team.
    C. the staffing limits.
    D. the changing needs of the patient.

12. It is important that the nursing assistant review the plan of care each day to
    A. see what information on the plan has changed.
    B. make suggestions, as a way to contribute to the plan.
    C. identify goals the patient is achieving.
    D. all of the above.

13. The plan of care will influence how the nursing assistant
    A. organizes his work.
    B. plans his work.
    C. observes and reports the patient's activities.
    D. all of the above.

14. The nursing assistant is responsible for
    A. gathering data objectively.
    B. reporting data in a timely manner.
    C. documenting the care given to the patient.
    D. all of the above.

15. The patient must be identified by _____ before preparing to transfer him.
    A. asking the family or visitors who he is
    B. asking him if he is the one to be transferred
    C. checking the identification bracelet
    D. calling the doctor

16. The nursing assistant should be aware that some patients will be _____ that they must be transferred to another facility or even to another unit.
    A. alarmed
    B. angry
    C. anxious
    D. all of the above

17. The nursing assistant can give the patient emotional support after transferring him by
    A. reassuring him that his family will find him eventually.
    B. telling him he shouldn't worry so much because he could be moved again tomorrow.
    C. telling him about other patients you have transferred today.
    D. reassuring him that his family and visitors will be given the new room number.

18. A common way to transfer the patient is
    A. on a wheelchair scale.
    B. on a draw sheet.
    C. on a stretcher or in a wheelchair.
    D. all of the above.

19. After the transfer, the immediate supervisor will want to know all of the following except
    A. the time of the transfer.
    B. the patient's reaction to the transfer.
    C. the number of patients discharged that day.
    D. observations of anything unusual.

20. If the patient is discharged to another health care facility,
    A. the patient may require a caregiver or nurse to accompany him.
    B. the nursing assistant will not be involved in this kind of transfer.
    C. an ambulance is never used.
    D. there will be no special instructions from the nurse.

21. Today, patients tend to have shorter convalescent periods at home than in the past.
    A. True
    B. False
    Correct Answer: _____

22. Teaching patients how to care for themselves at home is the responsibility of
    A. the nursing assistant only.
    B. the nurse only.
    C. the entire nursing team.
    D. the person who chooses to take on that responsibility.

23. The patient's family must be included in the discharge education process because
    A. it's nice to be included.
    B. the family may be the primary caregivers at home.
    C. they want to be included.
    D. they are paying the bill.

24. The best approach to discharge teaching is the
    A. partial approach.
    B. complete approach.
    C. holistic approach.
    D. discharge approach.

25. The discharge instructions will include
    A. detailed housekeeping instructions.
    B. detailed travel arrangements.
    C. details on diet, activity, and medications.
    D. information on how to discharge a patient.

26. Explanation of care in the home environment will include information on
    A. available transportation and elimination of hazards in the home.
    B. available housekeeping services.
    C. economic support agencies.
    D. all of the above.

27. The nursing assistant should ask the patient if he has the written discharge information before wheeling him off the floor.
    A. True
    B. False
    Correct Answer: _____ _____

28. It is the nursing assistant's responsibility to read and understand her institution's policies and procedures for _____ of the patient.
    A. admission
    B. discharge
    C. transfer
    D. all of the above

29. By following the plan of care, the nursing assistant will contribute to the nursing team's goal for quality patient care.
    A. True
    B. False
    Correct Answer: _____

COMPETENCY CHECKLIST 8-1: ADMITTING, TRANSFERRING, AND DISCHARING A PATIENT

ACTIVITY	S	U	COMMENTS
1. The student will demonstrate the correct method for:			
A. Admitting a patient			
B. Weighing and measuring the height of a patient			
C. Transferring a patient			
D. Discharging a patient			

THE PATIENT'S ENVIRONMENT

The following exercises will assist you to apply what you have read in Chapter 9, "The Patient's Environment." For each example, read the objective and use information you have read in Chapter 9 to answer the questions, complete the sentences, or label the diagrams.

EXERCISE 9-1

Objective: To recognize the definitions of words related to the patient's environment.

Directions: Place the letter of the correct definition next to the matching word from the word list.

Word List	Definitions
____ 1. alternating-pressure mattress	A. Capable of burning quickly and easily
____ 2. lamb's wool	B. A frame shaped like a barrel cut in half lengthwise and used to keep bed linens off a part of the patient's body
____ 3. equipment	C. A central place for storing supplies and equipment
____ 4. bedpan	D. A chair on wheels used to transport patients
____ 5. stretcher	E. A pad similar to an air mattress that can be placed beneath the patient to reduce pressure on the head, shoulders, back, heels, elbows, and bony prominences
____ 6. walker	F. The space for one patient, including the hospital bed, bedside table, chair, and other equipment
____ 7. patient lift	G. A tall pole, also called an IV pole, which attaches to a bed or is on rollers or casters; this pole is used to hold the containers or tubes needed, for example, during a blood transfusion

____ 8. Central Supply Department

____ 9. flammable

____ 10. patient unit

____ 11. specialty bed

____ 12. wheelchair

____ 13. bed cradle

____ 14. urinal

____ 15. emesis basin

____ 16. disposable equipment

____ 17. intravenous pole

____ 18. foot board

____ 19. bed board

____ 20. binders

H. Materials, tools, devices, supplies, furnishings, necessary things used to perform a task

I. A pan used by patients who must defecate or urinate while in bed

J. A portable container given to male patients in bed so they can urinate without getting out of bed

K. Equipment that is used one time only or for one patient only and then thrown away

L. A stable frame made of metal tubing used to support the unsteady patient while walking; the patient holds the walker while taking a step, moves it forward, and takes another step

M. A narrow rolling table with or without a mattress, or simply a canvas stretched over a frame, used to transport patients; the latter may also be called a litter or a gurney

N. A mechanical device with a sling seat used for lifting a patient into and out of such equipment as the hospital bed, bathtub, or wheelchair

O. A wide strip of lamb's hide with the fleece attached, or an imitation material, used to increase patient comfort

P. A bed that constantly changes pressure under the patient; used to minimize pressure points in the treatment or prevention of pressure ulcers

Q. A pan used for catching material that a patient spits out, vomits, or expectorates

R. Strips of heavy cotton cloth with Velcro fasteners; these are wrapped securely around the patient's body over the abdomen to give support and comfort following abdominal surgery

S. A small board placed upright at the foot of the bed and used to keep the patient's feet aligned properly to prevent foot drop

T. A large board placed beneath the mattress to provide additional support for patients with back, muscle, or bone problems

EXERCISE 9-2

Objective: To recognize important actions to take in accident prevention and reporting.

Directions: The five categories listed below (HFS, CFH, BP, HSH, RET) are about accident prevention and reporting. For each of the specific safety items listed below, select an appropriate category. You may select more than one category for each item.

HFS = home fire safety   HSH = home safety hazards
CFH = calling for help   RET = reporting an emergency by telephone
BP = burn prevention

Possible answers include:

_____ 1. If a fire occurs, get the patient out of the area.

_____ 2. The fire department emergency number is kept near the telephone

_____ 3. Cluttered hallways and walkways

_____ 4. Loose rugs that slip or do not have a nonskid backing

_____ 5. Avoid using flammable liquids

_____ 6. Check the temperature of water before using it on the patient.

_____ 7. Wet floor

_____ 8. Have handy the telephone number of the poison control center.

_____ 9. Give the name of the patient and identify your location, room number, or address.

_____ 10. Unstable furniture

_____ 11. Give your name first when you call.

_____ 12. Keep matches away from children and confused adults.

_____ 13. Sharp objects such as knives, razors, and hypodermic needles

_____ 14. Poisons (such as cleaning solutions)

_____ 15. Clearly state the problem: objectively state exactly what has happened or what help you need.

_____ 16. Faulty or uneven stairs or loose debris on stairs

_____ 17. Have the number of your home care supervisor near the telephone.

EXERCISE 9-3

Objective: To apply what you have learned about the patient's environment.

Directions: Circle the letter next to the word or statement that best completes the sentence or describes the sentence as true or false. If the sentence is false, draw a line through the incorrect part of the sentence and write the correction on the blank line.

1. Disposable equipment requires washing and disinfecting.
    A. True
    B. False
    Correct Answer: _____

2. When the nursing assistant is unfamiliar with the equipment used, he must ask for an inservice or
    A. must ask the patient how others have used it.
    B. make a wild guess and try to figure it out by himself.
    C. quickly try to get the equipment to work.
    D. review instructions prior to working with the item.

3. Disposable equipment may be reused by other patients if it is washed in hot soapy water.
    A. True
    B. False
    Correct Answer: _____

4. Nursing assistants usually can get disposable equipment from
    A. the cafeteria supply department.
    B. the dirty utility room.
    C. other patients' rooms.
    D. the Central Supply Department.

5. A primary goal is to make the patient feel
    A. comfortable in the hallway.
    B. comfortable in his environment.
    C. more important than other patients.
    D. busy and occupied after surgery.

6. The patient's room or unit is his environment when in the hospital or long-term care facility.
    A. True
    B. False
    Correct Answer: _____

7. If the patient has belongings from home, the nursing assistant
    A. should demonstrate respect for the articles.
    B. should borrow the articles if needed.
    C. should rearrange them to suit his own preferences.
    D. should instruct the family to take them back home.

8. The nursing assistant should create a
    A. safe environment for his patients.
    B. complex and busy environment for the patient.
    C. list of environmental rules for the patient and family to follow.
    D. risky environment to keep the patient alert to danger.
9. The unit should be arranged
    A. for the comfort of the nursing assistant.
    B. for the convenience of the patient.
    C. by the immediate supervisor only.
    D. in a complex and mazelike pattern.
10. A key word to remember when rearranging furniture is
    A. anticipation.
    B. drudgery.
    C. speed.
    D. obstacle course.
11. If the patient is right handed, place the call light near
    A. the doorway.
    B. the left ear.
    C. the telephone.
    D. the right hand.
12. A unit designed for a child is the same as for an adult.
    A. True
    B. False
    Correct Answer: _____
13. The two most important factors that will determine how a pediatric unit is arranged and the equipment that will be needed are
    A. the age of the child and the parents.
    B. the diagnosis only.
    C. the age of the nursing assistant.
    D. the age of the child and the reason for hospitalization.
14. If there is more than one unit in a room, draw curtains can be used for privacy.
    A. True
    B. False
    Correct Answer: _____

BEDMAKING

The following exercises will assist you to apply what you have read in Chapter 10, "Bedmaking." For each exercise, read the objective and use information you have read in Chapter 10 to answer the questions, complete the sentences, or label the diagrams.

EXERCISE 10-1

Objective: To apply what you have learned about the different methods of bedmaking.

Directions: Choose terms from the Word List to label the four methods of bedmaking in Figure 10-1. Then, next to each Practice Description, write the number of the correct method of bedmaking you would use.

Word List

occupied   postoperative   open   closed

FIGURE 10-1

1. _____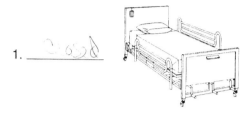

3. _postop_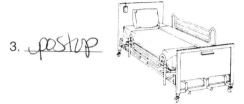

2. _open_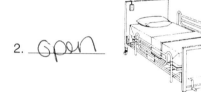

4. _occupied_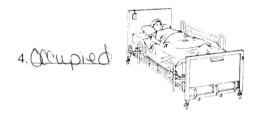

Practice Description

3 1. Mrs. O'Shea will be returning from surgery in the next two hours.

4 2. You have finished giving Mr. Garcia a complete bath. He is a stroke patient and is too weak to get out of bed.

2 3. Mrs. Chang is being ambulated in the hallway, so you decide to make her bed now.

1 4. Your patient has been discharged, the room and bed have been cleaned, and your immediate supervisor asks you to make the bed.

EXERCISE 10-2

Objective: To be able to correctly recall bedmaking guidelines.

Directions: Circle the letter next to the statement that best completes the sentence.

1. By fanfolding the top of the bed, you make it easier for the patient to
   A. roll out of bed in the morning.
   B. bathe himself.
   C. make his own bed.
   D. get back into the bed.

2. Shaking the bed linen
    A. can be done safely in the hallway.
    B. should not be done because it disturbs the doctors.
    C. should be done daily.
    D. spreads germs and should not be done.
3. When a cotton draw sheet is not available,
    A. you do not need to use one.
    B. re-use the one that was taken off earlier.
    C. use a large sheet which has been folded in half lengthwise.
    D. use a large sheet that has been folded in half widthwise.
4. Torn or damaged linen should
    A. be disposed of in red bags.
    B. be used to make the bed.
    C. be torn into strips and used for cleaning.
    D. be sent for repair according to the policy of your institution.
5. Wrinkles in the sheet
    A. promote good circulation by stimulating the skin.
    B. may be avoided by pulling the sheet tightly to smoothe it.
    C. can be removed by the patient lying on it for two hours.
    D. will not occur if it is made of cotton fabric.
6. You can save time and energy when making a bed if you
    A. get someone else to do it.
    B. stand either at the head or at the foot of the bed.
    C. make one side of the bed and then quickly crawl across to the other side.
    D. use good body mechanics to make as much of the bed as possible on one side before going to the other side.
7. The _____ side of a bed protector should never touch a patient's skin.
    A. cotton
    B. wet
    C. plastic
    D. white
8. A rubber or plastic bed protector can be used if it
    A. is clean.
    B. is covered by a cotton sheet.
    C. is dry.
    D. can be pulled tightly to remove all wrinkles.
9. Wrinkles in the sheets can
    A. make the patients sleep soundly.
    B. cause skin breakdown, leading to decubitus ulcers.
    C. be ignored.
    D. be removed by shaking them vigorously.

10. Taking extra linen into a patient's unit
   A. is a good idea because if it is not used it can be put back on the linen cart and used later for someone else.
   B. is a wasteful practice.
   C. makes the patient feel cared for.
   D. is convenient because you will have extra linen if you need it.

COMPETENCY CHECKLIST 10-1: BEDMAKING SKILLS

ACTIVITY	S	U	COMMENTS
1. Student correctly demonstrates the open method of bedmaking.			
2. Student correctly demonstrates the closed method of bedmaking.			
3. Student correctly demonstrates the postoperative method of bedmaking.			
4. Student correctly demonstrates the occupied method of bedmaking.			

HOME HEALTH CARE

The following exercises will assist you to apply what you have read in Chapter 11, "Home Health Care." For each exercise, read the objective and use information you have read in Chapter 11 to answer the questions, complete the sentences, or label the diagrams.

EXERCISE 11-1

Objective: To recognize and correctly spell words related to home health care.

Directions: Unscramble the words in the Word List at the left. Then circle the same words in the Word Search at the right.

Word List

1. EBD-BNDUO_____

2. FYAILM NTIU_____

3. NOGL RMTE_____

4. EARCVEGIR _____

5. MREENGCYE_____

6. MOEH LEHTHA _____

7. EIAD _____

8. EGRAHCSID _____

Word Search

B	E	D	B	O	U	N	D	C	E	P	B	E	D	X
A	L	E	S	G	Z	W	G	L	M	T	R	A	C	D
P	F	T	R	Z	A	C	A	B	E	S	V	X	D	L
G	A	B	X	T	L	Q	G	J	R	B	H	W	S	N
X	M	W	N	U	S	I	C	P	G	I	T	B	I	G
K	I	X	V	D	A	O	A	J	E	A	L	E	N	T
S	L	O	N	G	T	E	R	M	N	V	A	I	D	E
Q	Y	E	S	F	Y	Z	E	L	C	B	E	Y	C	X
L	U	I	R	T	Z	Y	G	E	Y	C	H	L	D	V
B	N	T	C	O	A	H	I	B	B	R	E	M	J	U
C	I	L	A	D	R	M	V	D	I	O	M	E	C	L
S	T	F	M	X	S	D	E	G	T	X	O	A	G	D
O	D	S	W	F	L	Z	R	D	B	C	H	F	S	O
D	I	S	C	H	A	R	G	E	O	A	S	T	W	P

EXERCISE 11-2

Objective: To be able to recognize the variety of important duties you will perform as a home health nursing assistant.

Directions: Place the correct letters next to the matching phrase. More than one set of letters may be selected for some of the phrases.

ADL = activities of daily living
C   = communication
CE   = care of the environment
IC   = infection control
N   = nutrition
PC   = personal care

PMT = positioning, moving, transporting the patient
SKC = skin care
SP   = special procedures
SPC = specimen care
VS   = vital signs

Answers may vary; possible answers include:

_____ 1. Informing the patient of procedures you perform
_____ 2. Washing the bathtub before and after use
_____ 3. Recording intake and output
_____ 4. Washing the dishes used to prepare the meals
_____ 5. Keeping the patient's skin clean and dry
_____ 6. Making the patient's bed and changing the linen as needed
_____ 7. Changing simple dressings and applying nonmedicated ointment
_____ 8. Transporting the patient to the doctor's office
_____ 9. Assisting the patient to use a bedside commode
_____ 10. Application of an elastic bandage to the patient's leg
_____ 11. Grocery shopping for the patient
_____ 12. Helping the patient brush his teeth and get dressed
_____ 13. Taking the temperature, pulse, respirations, and blood pressure
_____ 14. Positioning the patient in the bed
_____ 15. Using good hand washing skills and wearing disposable gloves
_____ 16. Performing range-of-motion exercises
_____ 17. Make an accurate record of duties performed for the patient
_____ 18. Washing the patient's clothing and linens
_____ 19. Cooking and preparing nutritious meals for the patient
_____ 20. Applying a binder to the patient

EXERCISE 11-3

Objective: To demonstrate appropriate responses to family situations.

Directions: Read the situation description and then choose the appropriate response.

1. You are assigned to provide home care three hours a day for a patient who is terminally ill with advanced lung cancer. She and her husband smoke heavily each time you are there. You are a nonsmoker and do not like being exposed to the smoke. Although the doctor has encouraged the family to *not* smoke, they choose to continue. **What would you do?**

    A. You continue to inform them about the dangers of smoking.

    B. You repeatedly inform them of your dislike of smoking.

    C. You tell them, "It's me or the cigarettes! Make your choice!"

    D. You arrange to have the husband leave the room when he smokes, and you leave the room when the patient smokes.

2. You are uneasy around your home care patient's pet, a large dog. Each time you visit the home, he follows you around, growling occasionally, and watches you closely as you care for the patient. **What would you do?**

    A. Bring the dog a bone to occupy him each time you visit.

    B. Take him by the collar and put him outside.

    C. Explain how you feel to the patient, and ask that the dog be put in another room or outside when you visit.

    D. Ignore the dog and pretend it doesn't bother you.

3. The family members begin to argue with each other about whose turn it is to do the laundry for your patient. **What would you do?**

    A. Since you know who should be doing the laundry, you point him out to the group.

    B. Offer to do the laundry for the family.

    C. Continue to care for the patient and do not get involved in the argument.

    D. Ask the family to stop arguing.

4. You notice that your home care patient's family members use the same drinking glass each time they get a drink of water. **What would you do?**

    A. You tell them about all the colds and flu they can catch from this practice.

    B. When you are there, you switch to a clean glass after they leave the room, so that the next person will not use a contaminated glass.

    C. You rush over and wash the glass after each use.

    D. You notify the home health nurse so that she can do some health teaching with the family on this issue.

5. When working at a patient's home, you observe that it is very dusty, dirty, and cluttered. **What would you do?**

    A. You decide to be nice and stay late one day to clean the entire house so that it meets your standards.

    B. You offer to clean up the mess for pay.

    C. You ignore the condition of the house and focus on the patient.

    D. You call up some of the patient's relatives and ask them to clean the house before your next visit.

6. You notice that the locked security grates over all the windows would not allow escape in case of a fire. **What would you do?**
   A. Talk to the family about a plan of escape in case of fire.
   B. Bring this situation to the attention of your supervisor immediately.
   C. Talk to the family about the danger posed by the grates on the windows.
   D. All of the above.

EXERCISE 11-4

Objective: To recognize the definitions of words related to the nursing assistant and home health care.

Directions: Place the letter of the correct definition next to the matching word from the word list.

Word List		Definitions	
____	1. time/travel record	A.	Unable to get out of bed
____	2. short-term intermittent skilled nursing care	B.	The family member or significant other who is taking the major responsibility for care of the patient
____	3. sterilize	C.	Getting all of one's duties completed in an organized fashion within a designated work period
____	4. flammable	D.	A group brought together by shared needs, interests, and mutual concern for the well-being of all its members
____	5. efficiency	E.	Capable of burning quickly and easily
____	6. bed-bound	F.	A liquid food prescribed for an infant containing most required nutrients
____	7. infection control	G.	The care of patients with terminal conditions who choose to remain at home until their death
____	8. punctuality	H.	Restraining or curbing the spread of microorganisms
____	9. family unit	I.	The care of chronically ill patients who are unable to care for themselves and live alone or have limited family support
____	10. microorganism	J.	Arriving at one's planned destination on time
____	11. caregiver	K.	A living thing so small it cannot be seen with the naked eye but only through a microscope
____	12. hospice care	L.	A duty or obligation; that for which one is accountable
____	13. responsibility	M.	The care provided to acutely ill patients or those with an exacerbated illness, with the purpose of educating the patients to become independent in self-care and functional ability

_____14. formula

_____15. long-term
        supportive care

N. Destroying all microorganisms

O. A record or log describing how time is spent in a patient's home and/or an account of the time it took to and from the patient's home or running errands

EXERCISE 11-5

Objective: To apply what you have learned about home health care.

Directions: Circle the letter next to the word or statement that best completes the sentence or describes the sentence as true or false. If the sentence is false, draw a line through the incorrect part of the sentence and write the correction on the blank line.

1. Helpful personal qualities of the home health aide are all of the following except
    A. the ability to be a self-starter.
    B. dependability and punctuality.
    C. an ethical approach to patient care.
    D. musical ability.

2. By not discussing the patient's condition with your family you show
    A. respect for the privacy of your patient.
    B. respect for the confidentiality of the patient.
    C. both A and B.
    D. a lack of interest in your patient.

3. In your role as a home health care aide, it is important to maximize your time by
    A. balancing time and money.
    B. balancing patient preferences with travel distances.
    C. driving at high speeds, when necessary, to be on time.
    D. leaving your patient assignment early, so that you can be on time for the next patient.

4. If you are delayed _____, you must call the patient to set a new arrival time.
    A. more than 30 minutes
    B. more than 45 minutes
    C. more than 2 days
    D. for any amount of time

5. The number one complaint of home health care aides is lack of punctuality by the patient.
    A. True
    B. False
    Correct Answer: _____

6. As a member of the health care team, you are expected to maintain _____ in the home.
   A. the status quo
   B. a sense of humor
   C. complete silence
   D. a professional attitude

7. While working in the home, you are part of the health care team, but an important difference is that you will usually not have another member of the team
   A. to whom you can refer problems.
   B. to whom you can speak if you have questions.
   C. physically present in the home with you while you care for the patient.
   D. to act as a supervisor.

8. An example of demonstrating honesty and accuracy when handling the patient's money is to
   A. attach all receipts to the shopping list.
   B. mix it with your own money.
   C. simply tell the patient what you have spent, because you know he has a good memory.
   D. keep the loose change for yourself.

9. In most cases, the goal of patient care in the home is to promote increasing dependence of the patient on the home health aide.
   A. True
   B. False
   Correct Answer: _____

10. The home health aide is responsible for making the first home evaluation and developing the plan of care to be followed by caregivers.
    A. True
    B. False
    Correct Answer: _____

11. The discharge planning process requires communication with the home health care team by all members except
    A. the patient.
    B. the banker.
    C. the home health aide.
    D. the nurse.

12. It is important that all team members understand what the _____ are for each patient's plan of care.
    A. outcome prices
    B. outcome goals
    C. outcome costs
    D. insurance benefits

13. The home health aide must be alert to prevent accidents in the patient's home by_____ unsafe conditions.
    A. creating, berating, and aggregating
    B. improvising, supervising, and relating
    C. maintaining, prolonging, and inventing
    D. eliminating, preventing, and correcting

14. When all the outcome goals have been met, the patient will
    A. receive the bill.
    B. be cured.
    C. be hospitalized.
    D. be discharged from home care.

15. If you are not sure how long a baby's formula has been in the refrigerator,
    A. taste it yourself.
    B. boil it for ten minutes.
    C. leave it in there for another time.
    D. discard it and make fresh formula.

16. The use of boiled and then cooled water to make formula is important because boiling will kill the microorganisms in the water. These microorganisms may make the baby sick.
    A. True
    B. False
    Correct Answer: _____

17. There are several different kinds of formulas, but in all cases it is important to
    A. wash your hands, as well as the containers before opening them.
    B. read the instructions for preparation.
    C. shake all containers of liquid and concentrated formulas before opening.
    D. do all of the above.

18. Once formula is prepared it must be
    A. fed to the infant immediately.
    B. fed to the infant after boiling for ten minutes.
    C. kept refrigerated until ready to use.
    D. kept at room temperature.

19. The home health aide may have housekeeping responsibilities in addition to care of the patient.
    A. True
    B. False
    Correct Answer: _____

20. _____ is an inexpensive disinfectant found in most homes that can be used to clean sinks, bathtubs, and toilets.
    A. Isopropyl alcohol
    B. A mixture of vinegar and oil
    C. Baking soda and vinegar
    D. Laundry bleach

21. When preparing food for the patient, remember to consider
    A. your likes and dislikes.
    B. the cultural and religious preferences of the patient.
    C. special dietary restrictions the patient may have.
    D. both B and C.

22. It is best to arrange your visit during the mealtime hours if part of your duties are to
    A. eat three meals a day.
    B. bathe the patient only.
    C. do the laundry.
    D. prepare a meal and record the amount eaten.
23. To be a self-starter means to be able to
    A. carry out duties with much assistance.
    B. accomplish only tasks you started yourself.
    C. work independently and effectively.
    D. start working only when by yourself.
24. If a patient has no toothpaste or denture cleaner, you may use _____ in its place.
    A. salt
    B. handsoap
    C. baking soda
    D. vinegar
25. When you show respect for the cultural beliefs and customs of the patient and his family, you
    A. make them feel valued as individuals.
    B. will make them like you.
    C. will change their daily habits.
    D. will make them happy.

COMPETENCY CHECKLIST 11-1: INFANT CARE

ACTIVITY	S	U	COMMENTS
1. The student will demonstrate the proper procedure for sterilizing tap water.			
2. The student will demonstrate the proper procedure for sterilizing bottles, nipples, and caps.			
3. The student will demonstrate the proper procedure for preparing:			
a. Ready-to-feed formula			
b. Powdered formula			
c. Concentrated liquid formula			

PERSONAL CARE OF THE PATIENT

The following exercises will assist you to apply what you have read in Chapter 12, "Personal Care of the Patient." For each exercise, read the objective and use information you have read in Chapter 12 to answer the questions, complete the sentences, or label the diagrams.

EXERCISE 12-1

Objective: To be able to apply the correct meaning of words used to describe the personal care of patients.

Directions: Choose from the Word List the correct word that matches the definition.

Word List

dentures   bedpan   self-care   urinal   ADL   commode
urinate   flow sheet   oral hygiene   defecate   incontinence
fracture pan

List of Definitions

1. To rid the body of waste matter from the bowels. _____
2. A portable container given to male patients so they can urinate without getting out of bed. _____
3. Cleanliness of the mouth. _____
4. To discharge urine from the body. _____
5. A checklist or chart for recording the activities of daily living. _____
6. The inability to control the bowels or bladder. _____
7. Activities or care tasks performed by the patient. _____
8. A pan used by patients who must defecate or urinate while in bed. _____
9. The activities or tasks usually performed every day, such as toileting, washing, eating, or dressing. _____

10. A movable chair enclosing a bedpan or having an opening that can fit over a toilet. _____

11. Artificial teeth. _____

12. A shallow bedpan used by patients with mobility limitations._____

EXERCISE 12-2

Objective: To recognize and correctly spell words related to helping the patient take a shower.

Directions: Unscramble the words in the Word List at the left. Then circle these same words in the Word Search at the right.

Word List

1. HICAR_____

2. THAB LOSTEW _____

3. PASO_____

4. WASHPEROC_____

5. HASTLOWCH_____

6. HBTA TMA _____

7. NECLA NOWG_____

8. FEDINISTANTC NOISTULO _____

_____

9. NAYLDUR AGB _____

10. ABLEDSIPOS SOGLEV_____

Word Search

R	U	N	O	D	P	G	S	I	T	W	R	Y	J	U	P
O	K	Y	D	I	P	R	U	P	Z	I	W	T	R	A	A
N	N	O	T	S	U	W	Q	P	B	A	C	T	S	U	S
J	C	H	A	I	R	Q	J	E	F	Z	R	T	Z	T	K
F	A	U	P	N	L	L	I	A	M	J	B	B	U	W	E
L	T	K	J	F	O	G	J	U	O	D	B	U	D	C	Z
W	H	T	H	E	V	C	K	U	M	A	A	D	R	A	N
W	A	S	H	C	L	O	T	H	H	D	T	B	A	T	U
A	J	O	I	T	I	C	O	U	T	C	H	R	T	D	P
L	K	I	K	A	A	T	W	O	K	L	T	A	I	C	J
A	O	A	S	N	M	H	E	L	P	E	O	K	T	G	B
U	T	Z	O	T	O	B	R	E	A	A	W	E	A	J	C
N	O	B	A	S	I	B	I	W	R	N	E	S	N	T	D
D	I	S	P	O	S	A	B	L	E	G	L	O	V	E	S
R	U	N	N	L	J	T	H	E	K	O	S	X	Y	Z	Z
Y	Q	W	H	U	O	H	S	H	O	W	E	R	C	A	P
B	I	D	E	T	O	M	P	T	I	N	K	U	W	T	J
A	U	U	N	I	O	A	A	A	D	T	J	W	A	T	T
G	Y	M	U	O	U	T	S	M	E	O	Q	T	Y	O	S
O	T	P	U	N	T	I	T	E	L	W	P	T	Q	T	V

EXERCISE 12-3

Objective: To recognize when to discuss a change in patient condition or activity with your immediate supervisor. Example: Patient requires a change in his bathing procedure.

Directions: For each of the situations described below, identify the *change* in bathing procedure you think should be considered and discussed with your immediate supervisor. Place the correct letters next to the situation described.

CBB = complete bed bath   PBB = partial bed bath
TB = tub bath   S = shower

_____ 1. Mr. Thompson has had a partial bed bath ordered for the last two days. He will be discharged soon, and he walks to the bathroom and in the hallway with assistance. He tells you he usually takes showers at home.

_____ 2. Mrs. James will be going home tomorrow with her new baby. Yesterday, she received a partial bed bath. She is able to use the bathroom and dress herself with no difficulty today.

_____ 3. Mrs. Sun, a new nursing home resident, tells you that at home she liked to take tub baths. You check your list and see that you have been assigned to have her take a shower.

_____ 4. You are assigned to give Mr. Sims a partial bath. You notice that he does not wash himself thoroughly and complains of being very tired today.

_____ 5. Mrs. James likes to walk in her bare feet and has to be frequently reminded to put on her slippers. Her feet and toenails are quite dirty, and she has many callouses. She says that at home she likes to put a chair in the tub to sit on while she soaks her feet and washes. She has been taking partial bed baths.

EXERCISE 12-4

Objective: To apply what you have learned about giving personal care to a patient.

Directions: Circle the letter next to the statement that best completes the sentence or describes the sentence as true or false. If the sentence is false, draw a line through the incorrect part of the sentence and write the correction on the blank line.

1. Patient care must be unhurried and _____ to meet each patient's special needs.
   A. uninterrupted
   B. fast
   C. personalized
   D. worthwhile

2. A patient scheduled for surgery should
   A. brush his teeth after eating.
   B. have mouth care done.
   C. never have mouth care done within one hour of the operation.
   D. cancel his mouth care.

3. Always wear _____ when giving a patient mouth care.
   A. a mask
   B. a raincoat and boots
   C. disposable gloves
   D. a gown

4. Patients who are ordered to be on _____ should be encouraged to do as much as possible for themselves.
   A. self-care
   B. your care
   C. medicare
   D. patient care

5. Bath water should never be changed once you have started the bath.
   A. True
   B. False
   Correct Answer: _____

6. Perineal care is specific care given to the
   A. arms and legs.
   B. periorbital arches.
   C. ears and mouth.
   D. external genitalia and rectal area.

7. If the patient's fingernails or toenails need trimming,
   A. follow the policy of your institution regarding care of patient's nails.
   B. tell them to cut their nails.
   C. soak them in warm water.
   D. do nothing because this is not part of personal care.

8. Giving the patient hair care will make him
   A. hungry and tired.
   B. slim and trim.
   C. look better and feel better.
   D. want to go home.

9. Before shaving a patient's face,
   A. get advice from his wife.
   B. get permission from the patient and your immediate supervisor.
   C. make sure he is sleeping.
   D. wait until he is eating breakfast.

10. Incontinent patients should be checked to see if they are clean and dry only at the beginning and at the end of each shift.
    A. True
    B. False
    Correct Answer: _____

11. Decubitus ulcers can result if the patient's skin is not kept clean and dry.
    A. True
    B. False
    Correct Answer: _____

12. A foot rub is an important part of the daily care of the patient.
    A. True
    B. False
    Correct Answer: _____

13. Each person is to be treated
    A. as if he were family.
    B. according to the flow sheet.
    C. to a reward if he follows orders.
    D. as an individual.

14. Your observations while helping patients are important to other members of the health care team.

   A. True
   B. False
   Correct Answer: _____

15. Providing personal care of the patient in a skillful manner will

   A. take too much time.
   B. prevent avoidance of ADLs.
   C. increase his comfort and well-being.
   D. decrease his appetite.

COMPETENCY CHECKLIST 12-1: PERSONAL CARE

ACTIVITY	S	U	COMMENTS
1. Student correctly states the steps involved in:			
a. early morning care			
b. morning care			
c. afternoon care			
d. evening care			
2. Student correctly demonstrates oral hygiene:			
a. mouth care			
b. denture care			
3. Student correctly demonstrates how to bathe a patient:			
a. complete bed bath			
b. partial bed bath			
c. tub bath			
d. shower			
4. Student correctly demonstrates how to give perineal care:			
a. male perineal care			
b. female perineal care			
5. Student correctly demonstrates how to care for nails and feet:			
a. foot care for the elderly and diabetic patient			
b. routine foot care			
6. Student correctly demonstrates how to give a back rub:			
a. routine care			
b. special care			

COMPETENCY CHECKLIST 12-1: PERSONAL CARE *(continued)*

ACTIVITY	S	U	COMMENTS
7. Student correctly demonstrates how to change a patient's gown:			
a. routine change			
b. change when arm injured or patient has I.V.			
8. Student correctly demonstrates how to give hair care:			
a. washing the hair			
b. combing the hair			
9. Student correctly demonstrates how to shave a patient's beard:			
a. using a safety razor			
b. using an electric razor			
10. Student correctly demonstrates how to meet patient's elimination needs:			
a. offering bedpan			
b. offering urinal			
c. offering commode			
d. incontinent patient care			

CORE ELEMENTS OF PERSONAL CARE

1. Wash hands and wear gloves.
2. Provide privacy.
3. Meet patient's individual needs.
4. Care is unhurried.
5. Provide safety.
6. Follow all steps of the procedure.

EMERGENCY CARE

The following exercises will assist you to apply what you have read in Chapter 13, "Emergency Care." For each exercise, read the objective and use information you have read in Chapter 13 to answer the questions, complete the sentences, or label the diagrams.

EXERCISE 13-1

Objective: To recognize and correctly spell words related to emergency care.

Directions: Fill in the missing letters to correctly spell the 12 words listed below. The total number of letters is listed next to each word.

1. _ MER _ _ _ CY (9)
2. H _ _ _ RRH _ GE (10)
3. S _ _ CK (5)
4. F _ _ T A _ _ (8)
5. _ TRO _ E (6)
6. C _ RDIO _ _ LMON _ _ Y (15)
7. CA _ _ I _ C ARR _ _ _ (13)
8. RES _ _ _ ITA _ _ ON (13)
9. _ _ RDI _ V _ _ _ _ LAR (14)
10. P _ _ SO _ (6)
11. S _ _ Z _ _ E (7)
12. _ N _ _ HYL _ _ T _ C (12)

EXERCISE 13-2

Objective: To recognize the symptoms of shock.

Directions: Draw a line to connect the correct type of shock that matches the cause.

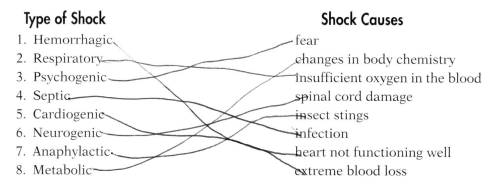

Type of Shock	Shock Causes
1. Hemorrhagic	fear
2. Respiratory	changes in body chemistry
3. Psychogenic	insufficient oxygen in the blood
4. Septic	spinal cord damage
5. Cardiogenic	insect stings
6. Neurogenic	infection
7. Anaphylactic	heart not functioning well
8. Metabolic	extreme blood loss

EXERCISE 13-3

Objective: To apply what you have learned about emergency care.

Directions: Circle the letter next to the word or statement that best completes the sentence or describes the sentence as true or false. If the sentence is false, draw a line through the incorrect part of the sentence and write the correction on the blank line.

1. Before you take any action in an emergency, you must determine all of the following except:
   A. What is the problem or emergency?
   B. Is there anyone available to help you?
   C. What must be done immediately to maintain life for the person in crisis?
   D. Do you, the nursing assistant, recognize the victim?
2. The emergency plan for home care patients should contain the telephone numbers for all of the following except
   A. fire rescue squads.
   B. emergency pedicure services.
   C. poison control center.
   D. physicians.
3. Guidelines for assisting a victim in an emergency do not include
   A. bleeding control.
   B. preventing further injury or harm.
   C. preventing shock.
   D. preventive care.

4. You may be called upon to perform _____ until medical help arrives.
   A. OBRA
   B. RACE
   C. PASS
   (D.) CPR

5. The _____ maneuver is used to dislodge an object and open the airway of a choking victim.
   A. karate
   B. choking
   (C.) Heimlich
   D. "last chance"

6. Placing your hands in the wrong position while doing chest compressions
   A. can improve the circulation.
   B. strengthens your hands.
   C. is not a major problem.
   (D.) can cause broken ribs and other problems for the victim.

7. Deliver 15 compressions to each breath during CPR.
   A. True
   B. False
   Correct Answer: _____ 5 Rcomp. / 2 Breaths

8. Deliver a compression rate of 80–100 for adult victims during CPR.
   (A.) True
   B. False
   Correct Answer: _____

9. A _____ is an episode, either partial or generalized, that may include alteration of consciousness, body movements, and convulsions.
   (A.) seizure
   B. stroke
   C. shock
   D. hemorrhage

10. A _____ is a site where a main artery lies near the surface of the body, directly over a bone.
    A. vein
    B. airway
    (C.) artery
    (D.) pressure point

11. _____ can be a sign of internal bleeding.
    (A.) Dilated pupils
    B. Extreme hunger
    C. Slow pulse
    D. Headache

12. Tissue damage caused by _____ is a burn.
    A. ice
    B. snow
    (C.) heat
    D. wind

13. Complications of a burn may include
 A. infection, shock, growth.
 B. pain, death, infection.
 C. promotion, infection, death.
 D. death, tanning, sleepiness.

14. Pale, moist, and cold skin may be a sign of
 A. death.
 B. birth.
 C. postshower syndrome.
 D. internal bleeding.

15. Internal bleeding can be accompanied by vomiting of
 A. breakfast.
 B. blood that looks like coffee grounds.
 C. blood that is greenish.
 D. blood that resembles tea.

16. Loss of _____ and body _____ is a complication of burns.
 A. milk, image
 B. heat, temperature
 C. heat, fluids
 D. heat, flexibility

17. A _____ is any substance that is toxic to the body.
 A. vitamin
 B. mineral
 C. radical
 D. poison

18. When assisting the patient who has been poisoned, you should do all of the following except
 A. check the mouth for burns.
 B. look for a container from which the poison may have come.
 C. note the odors on the person's breath.
 D. immediately induce vomiting.

19. After calling for medical assistance, a poisoning victim can be left alone.
 A. True
 B. False
 Correct Answer: _Never leave alone_

20. The regional poison control center is a good source of help in situations where the patient has been severely burned.
 A. True
 B. False
 Correct Answer: _____

21. If the person who has been poisoned is unconscious, give fluids by mouth to minimize the effect.
 A. True
 B. False
 Correct Answer: _Nothing_

22. The interruption of the blood supply to the heart muscle is called a
    _____

    A. muscle cramp.
    B. heart attack.
    C. pneumothorax.
    D. Heimlich episode.

23. The most important factor in successful resuscitation is the opening of
    the airway.

    A. True
    B. False

    Correct Answer: _____

24. If you suspect that a person has had a stroke, give only small bites of food
    immediately.

    A. True
    B. False

    Correct Answer: _____NO food or drink_____

25. When a person is having a seizure, you should protect him from injury and
    maintain a _____ airway.

    A. closed
    B. patent
    C. fluid
    D. obstructed

THE HUMAN BODY

The following exercises will assist you to apply what you have read in Chapter 14, "The Human Body." For each exercise, read the objective and use information you have read in Chapter 14 to answer the questions, complete the sentences, or label the diagrams.

EXERCISE 14-1

Objective: To be able to apply the correct meaning of words used to name tissues of the body.

Directions: Choose the correct word(s) from the Word List to complete the sentences.

Word List

muscle tissue	nerve tissue	connective tissue
epithelial tissue	cardiac muscle tissue	blood and lymph tissue
striated muscle tissue	smooth muscle tissue	tissues

1. Skin, linings of the intestines and linings of the glands and organs are examples of ___epithilial___ .
2. The function of ___Connective___ is to connect, support, cover or line, and pad or protect the body.
3. ___Muscle___ makes body movement possible.
4. The smooth, involuntary muscles made up of ___Cardiac___ keep the heart beating.
5. Muscles that can be moved with a conscious effort are made up of ___Striated___ .
6. ___Nerve___ carries impulses to and from the brain, spinal cord, and other parts of the body.
7. The tissue that has single cells and flows through vessels is known as ___Blood & lymph___

8. The dilation of such structures as the pupil of the eye and blood vessels is made possible by means of ___smooth___ .

9. ___tissues___ are groups of the same type of cells that work together.

EXERCISE 14-2

Objective: To be able to correctly describe cells and their functions.

Directions: Select the word(s) from the Word List to complete the sentences below.

Word List

building blocks	microscope	existed	living
oxygen	water	reproduce	

1. The cells are the fundamental ___building blocks___ of all living matter.
2. Cells can be seen only under the ___microscope___ .
3. Cells use ___water___ to transport substances.
4. Most living cells grow and ___reproduce___ themselves.
5. Cells use ___oxygen___ to break down food.
6. Cells are the ___living___ parts of organisms.
7. Cells come from cells that have already ___existed___ .

EXERCISE 14-3

Objective: To recognize and correctly spell words that name anatomical positions.

Directions: Unscramble the words in the Word List on the left. Then circle these same words in the Word Search at the right.

Word List

1. FORINERI ___inferior___
2. EPDE ___Dep___
3. LADSOR ___Dorsal___
4. RECAFUSPILI ___Superficial___
5. EROSIPUR ___Superior___
6. SORTERPIO ___posterior___
7. TANERORI ___Anterior___

Word Search

R	J	I	W	T	S	T	T	O	S	U	N
Q	W	T	L	D	E	E	P	S	U	T	U
D	O	R	S	A	L	W	A	I	P	R	M
I	E	D	U	N	D	A	C	T	E	V	B
P	P	O	S	T	E	R	I	O	R	J	E
P	S	U	P	E	R	F	I	C	I	A	L
I	N	F	E	R	I	O	R	A	O	K	S
D	U	M	P	I	T	A	L	L	R	O	T
I	T	I	W	O	J	A	M	M	S	T	W
O	J	O	L	R	I	T	U	V	E	Q	U

EXERCISE 14-4

Objective: To recognize and be able to correctly spell the names of various organs of the human body.

Directions: Label the diagram in Figure 14-1 with the correct words from the Word List below.

Word List

heart	lung	kidney
brain	uterus	liver
bladder	stomach	small intestine
large intestine	ovary	testicles

FIGURE 14-1

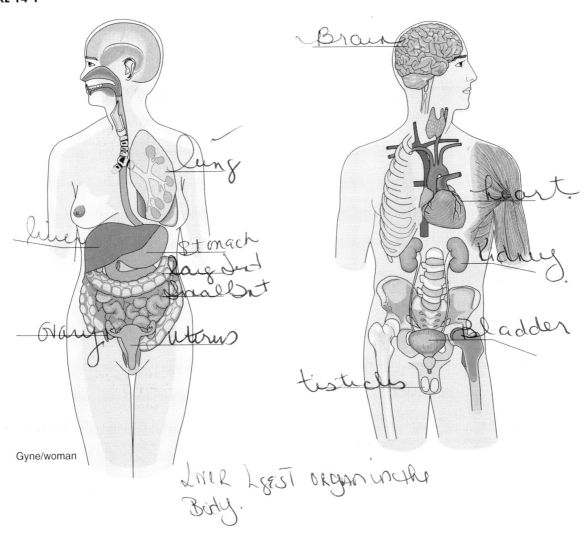

Gyne/woman

Liver Lgest organ in the Body.

EXERCISE 14-5

Objective: To apply your understanding of how the body cells, tissues, organs, and systems relate to each other.

Directions: Label the diagram in Figure 14-2 with the correct words from the Word List. Place the words in the *order of their complexity.*

Word List

organs   cells   systems   tissues

FIGURE 14-2

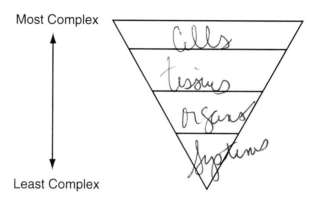

Most Complex

Least Complex

EXERCISE 14-6

Objectives: To apply what you have learned about the human body.

Directions: Circle the letter next to the word or statement that best completes the sentence or describes the sentence as true or false. If the sentence is false, draw a line through the incorrect part of the sentence and write the correction on the blank line.

1. The body systems cannot work by themselves and
   A. are dependent upon each other.
   B. so must borrow help from tissues.
   C. are independent of each other.
   D. let you know by complaining often.
2. The digestive system takes in and
   A. absorbs nutrients at night.
   B. absorbs daylight.
   C. absorbs nutrients as waste.
   D. absorbs nutrients and eliminates wastes.
3. An example of the integumentary system is
   A. the kidney.
   B. the heart.
   C. the brain.
   D. the skin.

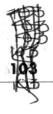

4. The urinary system controls activities of the body.
   A. True
   B. False
   Correct Answer: _____ Nervous _____

5. An organ of the respiratory system is the
   A. larynx.
   B. spleen.
   C. pancreas.
   D. thymus.

6. The integumentary system is the second and third line of defense against infection.
   A. True
   B. False
   Correct Answer: _____ First line _____

7. The front of a person is referred to as the
   A. anterior side.
   B. posterior side.
   C. the frontal lobe.
   D. first side.

8. Groups of cells of the same type that work together to perform a particular function are called tissues.
   A. True
   B. False
   Correct Answer: _____

9. Organs that work together to perform similar tasks make up body systems.
   A. True
   B. False
   Correct Answer: _____

10. The human back, containing the spine, is called the
    A. anterior or upper side.
    B. posterior or under side.
    C. posterior or weak side.
    D. posterior or dorsal side.

GROWTH AND DEVELOPMENT

The following exercises will assist you to apply what you have read in Chapter 15, "Growth and Development." For each exercise, read the objective and use information you have read in Chapter 15 to answer the questions, complete the sentences, or label the diagrams.

EXERCISE 15-1

Objective: To be able to correctly match the chronological stage to the developmental stage of human growth and development.

Directions: From the Word List below, select and write the name of the developmental stage next to the matching time period on the Age List.

Word List

preschool	adolescent	toddler	older adult
school-age	young adult	infant	middle adult

Age List

5–12 years	adolesent	1–2 year(s)	Toddler
12–18 years	yong adult	18–40 years	middle Adult
65+ years	Older adult	2–5 years	preschoel
birth–1 year	Infant	40–64 years	older Adult

EXERCISE 15-2

Objective: To be able to recognize developmental skills and the tasks that illustrate them.

Directions: Place the correct letters next to the matching phrase.

CS = cognitive skill   SS = social skill   LS = language skill
GMS = gross motor skill   FMS = fine motor skill

_____ 1. A preschool child recognizes colors.
_LS_ 2. The school-age child defines words.
_____ 3. The older adult adjusts to retirement.
_____ 4. The young adult selects a career.
_____ 5. The infant vocalizes, squeals, and imitates sounds.
_____ 6. The toddler throws balls.
_____ 7. The infant rolls over, pulls to sit, crawls, and stands alone.
_____ 8. The school-age child draws a man having six parts.
_____ 9. The infant feeds himself crackers.
_____10. The toddler expresses needs or indicates wants without crying.

EXERCISE 15-3

Objective: To apply what you have learned about nursing assistant behaviors and patient age-specific considerations.

Directions: Match the letter of the developmental stage with the correct age-specific consideration. Select only one answer for each statement.

Developmental Stages List

A. Infant: Birth–1 year
B. Toddler: 1–2 year(s)
C. Preschool: 2–5 years
D. School-age: 5–12 years

E. Adolescent: 12–18 years
F. Young adult: 18–40 years
G. Middle adult: 40–64 years
H. Older adult: 65+ years

Age-specific Consideration

_____ 1. Place visually interesting objects where the child can observe them.
_____ 2. Explain procedures in simple words, describing only what the patient will see.
_____ 3. Describe how long children will have to undergo a painful procedure.
_____ 4. Keep small objects, which may cause choking, out of child's reach.
_____ 5. Patient may request that a family member be present to provide support in making a health care decision.
_____ 6. Remember that body image is very important at this stage.
_____ 7. Remember that they have many obligations, such as parenthood and the care of their parents.
_____ 8. They are often concerned about how illness will affect their lifelong goals.

EXERCISE 15-4

Objectives: To apply what you have learned about your role as a nursing assistant.

Directions: Circle the letter next to the statement that best completes the sentence or describes the sentence as true or false. If the sentence is false, draw a line through the incorrect part of the sentence and write the correction on the blank line.

1. Growth refers to the measurable physical changes human beings experience throughout their lives.
    A. True
    B. False
    Correct Answer: _____

2. Development refers to the accomplishment of, and the increase in, the ability to use skills that people acquire over their life span.
    A. True
    B. False
    Correct Answer: _____

3. Growth and development usually follow
    A. growth spurts.
    B. each other.
    C. stages.
    D. death.

4. Growth continues through all the stages of life, but it begins
    A. at the beginning.
    B. at conception.
    C. at once.
    D. with life skills.

5. The gain in weight of infants from birth to 1 year
    A. is predictable within parameters.
    B. helps the mother feel better.
    C. is a sign of problems.
    D. is not measurable.

6. One indicator of proper growth is detected by
    A. measuring the baby's feet.
    B. measuring the mother's feet.
    C. measuring the umbilical cord.
    D. measuring the circumference of the baby's head periodically.

7. Humans build on skills they have developed
    A. at a previous stage of development.
    B. while sleeping.
    C. from observing their parents.
    D. through a nursing assistant course.

8. Injuries such as strokes make it necessary to relearn skills from earlier stages of development.
   A. True
   B. False
   Correct Answer: _____

9. When people are happy, they often behave at a lower developmental stage than their chronological age would indicate.
   A. True
   B. False
   Correct Answer: _____

10. Nursing assistants' ability to relate appropriately to patients is dependent on
    A. their awareness of the impact illness can have on patients at each stage of growth and development.
    B. the patient's attitude.
    C. whether they study this chapter.
    D. their immediate supervisor.

THE MUSCULOSKELETAL SYSTEM AND RELATED CARE

The following exercises will assist you to apply what you have read in Chapter 16, "The Musculoskeletal System and Related Care." For each exercise, read the objective and use information you have read in Chapter 16 to answer the questions, complete the sentences, or label the diagrams.

EXERCISE 16-1

Objective: To recognize and be able to correctly spell the parts of the musculoskeletal system.

Directions: Label the diagram in Figure 16-1 with the correct word from the Word List below.

Word List

Muscles:

tibialis anterior	gastronemius	sartorius
rectus abdominus	quadriceps femoris	deltoid
pectoralis major	sternocleidomastoidius	biceps
tensor facia latae	peroneus longus	
abdominal muscle	intercostals	

Bones:

humerus	fibulla	clavicle	metacarpals
metatarsals	scapula	tibia	ribs
vertebrae	maxilla	radius	femur
sternum	frontal bone	pelvic bone	
cervical vertebrae	patella	ulna	
parietal	phalanges	mandible	

FIGURE 16-1

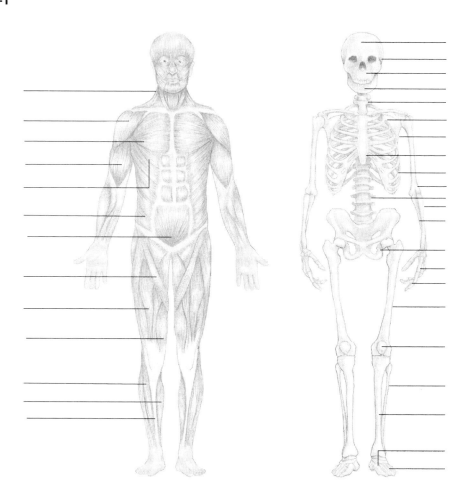

EXERCISE 16-2

Objective: To be able to name the category to which bones belong.

Directions: Draw a line to connect the bone with the correct category.

Category	Bone
Long Bones	vertebrae
Short Bones	ribs
Irregular Bones	phalanges
Flat Bones	femurs

EXERCISE 16-3

Objective: To correctly identify the types of joints of the human body.

Directions: Circle the words in the Word List below that identify the *major types of joints* of the human body.

Word List

shoulder	metatarsals	elbow	femur	wrist	mandible
radius	ankle	scapula	hip	radius	tibia
hinge	ball-and-socket	pivot	irregular joints of the spine		

EXERCISE 16-4

Objective: To recognize and correctly spell words that name the muscles of the body.

Directions: Unscramble the words in the Word List on the left. Then circle the same words in the Word Search at the right.

Word List

1. TIDOLED _Deltoid_
2. SUTSAV _Vastus_
3. ROTRASSUI _Sarto_
4. SEPCIB _Biceps_
5. LORTINCESTA _intercostal_
6. MIUSENROTSAG _Gastronomius_
7. CURTES _Rectus_
8. LABITISI _tibialis_

Word Search

D	A	B	D	O	M	U	N	I	L	U	Y	P	O	V	A	R
E	S	B	V	R	E	N	N	N	U	M	E	Q	H	A	A	E
L	A	K	O	P	M	Y	W	T	X	U	P	I	J	S	A	C
T	R	B	I	C	E	P	S	E	U	P	P	E	R	T	Q	T
O	T	H	G	A	S	R	R	R	C	N	E	M	I	U	S	U
I	O	W	N	I	M	C	I	C	E	R	H	I	V	S	Z	S
D	R	O	G	A	S	T	R	O	N	E	M	I	U	S		O
D	I	T	I	B	I	A	L	S	T	O	F	W	O	R	D	S
P	U	L	L	I	L	T	U	T	J	M	B	V	E	R	T	Y
H	S	H	U	M	P	A	A	A	A	D	A	F	A	L	L	X
M	A	H	T	I	B	I	A	L	I	S	T	T	L	E	L	A

EXERCISE 16-5

Objective: To recall common diseases and disorders of the orthopedic patient.

Directions: Complete the exercise sentences with the correct words from the Word List.

Word List

sprain	bone	simple fracture	joint dislocation
compound	Guillain-Barre	tuberculosis	muscular dystrophy
arthritis	spinal cord	poliomyelitis	trauma to spinal cord

1. An injury in which ligaments are partially torn is a _Sprain_
2. A fracture of a bone with *no* bone sticking out through the skin is called a _Simple fracture_
3. _Tuberculosis_ can be a disease of the bone; usually affects the lungs.
4. _Arthritis_ is known as a joint disease.
5. A _Joint Dislocation_ is the pulling out (displacement) of a bone end that forms part of a joint.
6. _Trauma_ can result in damage to the _____, causing paralysis of some area of the body.
7. A nervous system disease is the _Guillan Barre_ syndrome.
8. _Poliomielitis_ is a disease which is not often seen due to the use of preventive vaccines in babies and young children.
9. A disorder which can occur when muscles are immobile for several weeks or months is _Atrophy_.
10. A _Compound_ fracture is when the _____ is broken *and* there is an external wound or bone protruding through the skin.

EXERCISE 16-6

Objective: To apply what you have learned about the musculoskeletal system and related care.

Directions: Circle the letter next to the statement that best completes the sentence or describes the sentence as true or false. If the sentence is false, draw a line through the incorrect part of the sentence and write the correction on the blank line.

1. The healing of broken bones is a gradual process in which _____ is deposited at the fracture site.
   A. iron
   B. calcium
   C. glue
   D. blood

2. During each body movement, the skeletal system, the muscular system, the circulatory system, and the reproductive system are all interacting.
   A. True
   B. False
   Correct Answer: _____ nervous _____
3. Infection of a broken bone is more likely because
   A. of the size of the leg.
   B. when a bone is broken, the heart beats fast.
   C. poor blood supply to the bone means resistance to infection will be low.
   D. broken bones are painful.
4. The knee is an example of a _____ joint.
   A. rapid
   B. stiff
   C. painful
   D. hinge
5. The _____ connect muscle to bone.
   A. tendons
   B. tenderloins
   C. nerves
   D. synapses

   muscle to muscle is ligaments

6. Nursing assistants need to be familiar with orthopedic equipment such as
   A. splints, nasogastric tubes, and casts.
   B. casts, walkers, and thermometers.
   C. walkers, casts, and zippers.
   D. splints, casts, and walkers.
7. In the past, traction and bedrest were the methods of treatment for fractures, but today the emphasis is on
   A. low-fat diets.
   B. improved methods of surgery and extended hospital stays.
   C. lighter casting materials and early ambulation.
   D. shortened hospital stays and low-fat diets.
8. One of the benefits of early ambulation is fewer circulatory side effects.
   A. True
   B. False
   Correct Answer: _____
9. A device that replaces a bone or a joint is called a
   A. protrusion.
   B. prosthesis.
   C. proboscis.
   D. partition.
10. Some braces must be worn continually, and some are worn only when the patient is out of bed. Therefore, it is important to check the plan of care or ask your immediate supervisor for instructions if your patient is using a brace.
    A. True
    B. False
    Correct Answer: _____

11. Restricted _____ means that an orthopedic patient will need special skin care.

    A. permission
    B. mobility
    C. diet
    D. tolerance

12. The type of surgery a patient has will determine what kind of walker he should use.

    A. True
    B. False

    Correct Answer: _____

13. You should change the position of an immobile patient at least every 4 hours.

    A. True
    B. False

    Correct Answer: _____ 2 Hrs _____

14. A trapeze is a device that is suspended from an over-the-bed frame and allows the patient to

    A. receive better television reception.
    B. summon the nurse.
    C. swing forward and backward.
    D. move or lift himself more easily.

15. In the past, casts were made only out of plaster, a heavy material. Now casts are more often made of plastic or fiber-glass. These modern casts are lighter, allowing the patient to move more easily.

    A. True
    B. False

    Correct Answer: _____

16. Casts can become too tight after they are applied, causing the skin on either side of the cast edge to become blue or pale in color or hot to the touch.

    A. True
    B. False

    Correct Answer: _____ Cold to the touch _____

17. Any complaint of pain around, under, or near the cast must be reported immediately to the nurse or your immediate supervisor.

    A. True
    B. False

    Correct Answer: _____

18. Casts are in danger of becoming wet or soiled

    A. during the bath or while using the bedpan.
    B. after lunch when the patient goes swimming.
    C. when using the trapeze.
    D. while dressing the patient.

19. Casted extremities should be compared to uncasted extremities for
    A. changes in length.
    B. changes in flexibility.
    C. changes in size, color, and warmth.
    D. the presence of nodules.

20. An unusual odor coming from a cast could mean that
    A. fiber in the diet has been increased.
    B. it is ready to be removed.
    C. the extremity has healed.
    D. a pressure ulcer or infection is developing under the cast.

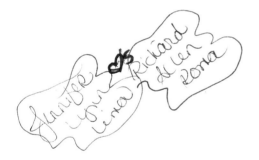

THE INTEGUMENTARY SYSTEM AND RELATED CARE

The following exercises will assist you to apply what you have read in Chapter 17, "The Integumentary System and Related Care." For each exercise, read the objective and use information you have read in Chapter 17 to answer the questions, complete the sentences, or label the diagrams.

EXERCISE 17-1

Objective: To recognize the definitions of words related to the integumentary system and related care.

Directions: Place the letter of the correct definition next to the matching word from the Word List below.

Word List		Definitions
1. epidermis	A.	Injuries resulting from the patient sliding against hard surfaces
2. atrophic skin	B.	An abnormality, either benign or cancerous, of the tissues of the body, such as a wound, sore, rash, boil, tumors, or growths
3. bony prominences	C.	Unable to control urine or feces
4. shear injuries	D.	The body system that includes the skin, hair, nails, and sweat and oil glands, that provides the first line of defense against infection, maintains body temperature, provides fluids, and eliminates wastes
5. lesion	E.	Also called bedsores; areas of the skin that become broken and painful; caused by continuous pressure on a body part and usually occur when a patient is kept in one position for a long period of time
6. incontinent	F.	The inner layer of skin
7. perineum	G.	Result from the skin remaining in place on top of a surface while the underlying structures, such as bone, slide downward

D 8. integumentary
       system
F 9. dermis
A 10. friction injuries

E 11. pressure ulcers
I 12. obese

H. Thin, fragile, less elastic skin frequently as-
    sociated with aging
I. Very overweight
J. The body area between the thighs (external
    genitalia and rectal area)
K. The outer layer or surface of the skin
L. Places where bones are close to the surface
    of the skin

EXERCISE 17-2

Objective: To identify important protective devices for the skin.

Directions: Read the following riddles carefully before writing the correct answer on the blank line.

1. This device helps to elevate an extremity off the bed. What is it? *Hint:* An alternative meaning goes well with coffee in the morning. _Donut_
2. This item is used to keep blankets off the legs and feet. What is it? *Hint:* An alternative meaning is a small bed for a baby. _Cradle_
3. This device prevents a serious deformity to the foot. What is it? *Hint:* An alternative meaning is something you would want to wear in the snow or rain. _____

EXERCISE 17-3

Objective: To recognize and correctly spell the structures of the skin.

Directions: Label the diagram in Figure 17-1 with the correct words from the Word List below.

Word List

sweat gland	epidermis	hair
sebaceous gland	dermis	fat
pores	blood vessel	nerve

FIGURE 17-1

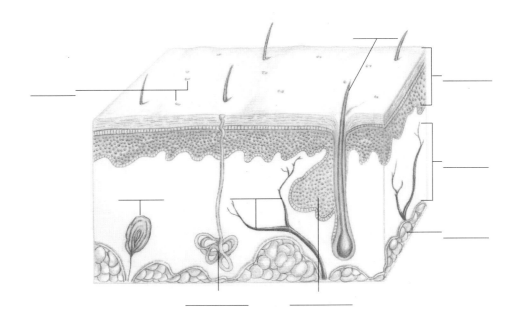

EXERCISE 17-4

Objective: To apply what you have learned about the integumentary system and related care.

Directions: Circle the letter of the word or phrase that best completes the sentence or describes the sentence as true or false. If the sentence is false, draw a line through the incorrect part of the sentence and write the correction on the blank line.

1. The _____ covers the entire body.
   A. dermis
   B. epidermis
   C. skin
   D. all of the above

2. _____ is responsible for the color of the skin.
   A. Dermis
   B. Epidermis
   C. Toner
   D. Pigment

3. The primary function of the skin is all of the following except to
   A. cover and protect underlying body structures from injury and invasion by microorganisms.
   B. provide an area for exchange of oxygen.
   C. help regulate body temperature.
   D. eliminate wastes through perspiration.

4. Serious health problems can cause _____ in the skin.
    A. changes
    B. improvement
    C. illumination
    D. healthy growth

5. Fungus is caused by _____ organisms.
    A. animal-like
    B. plant-like
    C. child-like
    D. solar-like

6. Chicken pox viruses can cause another painful skin disease called
    A. athlete's feet.
    B. pediculisis pedis.
    C. shingles.
    D. psoriasis.

7. As people age, the skin
    A. becomes more elastic.
    B. flakes off.
    C. grows thicker.
    D. becomes less elastic and more fragile.

8. People who are in shock will have skin that is more pale than usual.
    A. True
    B. False
    Correct Answer: _____

9. Loss of fat can make a person feel _____ even when room tem-
    peratures feel warm to others.
    A. thinner
    B. warmer
    C. cold
    D. sweaty

10. Pressure ulcers can develop because of prolonged pressure in an area, caus-
    ing a decrease in
    A. digestion.
    B. circulation.
    C. exercise.
    D. posture.

11. In addition to prolonged pressure, other reasons for decubitus ulcer for-
    mation are all of the following except
    A. a lack of cleanliness.
    B. moisture.
    C. material from wound drainage.
    D. body lotion applied in a circular motion after the bath.

12. All patients need to be observed to prevent pressure ulcer formation, all of the following are risk factors except:
    A. moist skin.
    B. mobility problems.
    C. good nutrition.
    D. numbness in a body part.

13. The pressure ulcer visible on the surface is often much smaller than the skin damage below the surface.
    A. True
    B. False
    Correct Answer: _____

14. The best place to check for signs of pressure are all of the following except
    A. the abdomen.
    B. the elbows.
    C. the hips.
    D. the sacrum.

15. The nursing assistant should report the first signs (redness) of an ulcer formation to the immediate supervisor.
    A. True
    B. False
    Correct Answer: _____

16. The type of pressure ulcer that is difficult to heal is
    A. a small ulcer.
    B. a moderate sized ulcer.
    C. a large ulcer.
    D. all of the above.

17. Friction/shear injuries can occur if
    A. the side rails are too high.
    B. the patient ambulates often.
    C. the gown is not tied tightly.
    D. the head of the bed is elevated too high.

18. To prevent friction/shear injuries,
    A. use a restraint on active patients.
    B. restrict bed movement.
    C. use a draw sheet to pull patients up in bed and for turning them.
    D. leave the patient on the bedpan for more than 20 minutes.

19. To prevent pressure between the legs when positioning the patient, use pillows.
    A. True
    B. False
    Correct Answer: _____

20. A patient using an eggcrate mattress will not develop a pressure ulcer.
    A. True
    B. False
    Correct Answer: _____

21. The feet must be kept in good alignment to prevent a serious deformity called
    A. alignment pox.
    B. athlete's foot.
    C. chin drop.
    D. foot drop.
22. Do not place an incontinent patient
    A. directly on the plastic side of the bed protector.
    B. directly on an incontinent pad.
    C. on a clean dry sheet.
    D. into a disposable diaper before sitting them in a chair.
23. The patient's position should be changed every 2 hours
    A. unless you are busy.
    B. unless they refuse to be repositioned.
    C. or less.
    D. during the day only.
24. If the patient's toenails need to be trimmed, the nursing assistant should
    A. trim them immediately.
    B. soak them before trimming them.
    C. notify the nurse.
    D. call the doctor.
25. In order to provide all the care a patient needs within a limited time frame, you must
    A. stop when tired.
    B. arrive earlier or work later than assigned.
    C. skip some of the work.
    D. plan the day efficiently

COMPETENCY CHECKLIST 17: SKIN CARE

ACTIVITY	S	U	COMMENTS
Student will demonstrate the correct method of providing safe skin cleansing for the incontinent patient.			

THE CIRCULATORY AND RESPIRATORY SYSTEMS AND RELATED CARE

The following exercises will assist you to apply what you have read in Chapter 18, "The Circulatory and Respiratory Systems and Related Care." For each exercise, read the objective and use information you have read in Chapter 18 to answer the questions, complete the sentences, or label the diagram.

EXERCISE 18-1

Objective: To recognize definitions of words related to the circulatory system and patient care.

Directions: Place the letter of the correct definition next to the matching word from the Word List.

Word List	Definitions
B 1. anemia	A. The continuous movement of blood through the heart and blood vessels to all parts of the body
I 2. heart	B. A shortage of red blood cells
E 3. blood pressure	C. A highly infectious disease that usually affects the lungs
A 4. circulation	D. Blood vessel that carries oxygenated blood away from the heart
L 5. vein	E. The force of the blood pushing against the walls of the blood vessels
C 6. tuberculosis	F. The heart, blood vessels, blood, and all organs that pump and carry blood and other fluids throughout the body
J 7. pulmonary	G. Pertaining to the heart
K 8. respiratory system	H. The liquid portion of the blood
D 9. artery	I. A four-chambered, hollow, muscular organ that lies in the chest cavity and pumps the blood through the lungs and into all parts of the body
F 10. circulatory system	J. Pertaining to the lungs

H 11. plasma

K. The group of body organs that carries on the body function of respiration; the system brings oxygen into the body and eliminates carbon dioxide

G 12. cardiac

L. Blood vessel that carries blood from parts of the body back to the heart

EXERCISE 18-2

Objective: To recognize and be able to correctly spell the names of various parts of the circulatory system.

Directions: Label the diagram in Figure 18-1 with the correct words from the word list below.

Word List

pulmonary capillaries	pulmonary veins	aorta (artery)
pulmonary arteries	systemic capillaries	venule
arteriole	capillaries	vena cavae (vein)

FIGURE 18-1

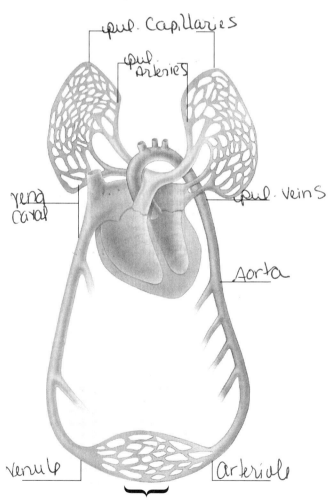

EXERCISE 18-3

Objective: To recognize and be able to correctly spell the names of various parts of the heart.

Directions: Label the diagram in Figure 18-2 with the correct words from the word list below.

Word List

superior vena cava   aorta   left atrium   right atrium
pulmonary artery   pulmonary veins   right ventricle
inferior vena cava   left ventricle   epicardium (outer covering)
myocardium (muscle)   pulmonary artery   pulmonary veins

FIGURE 18-2

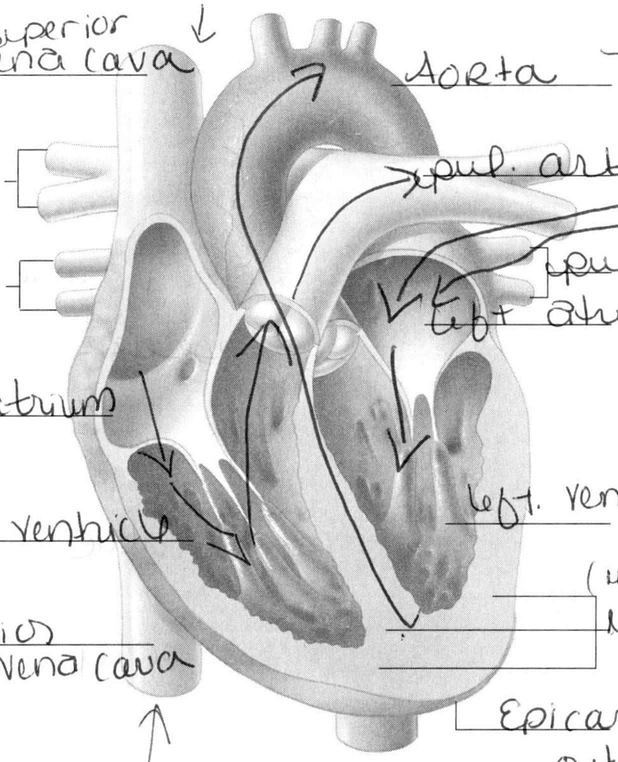

[handwritten annotations on heart diagram:]
upper Body
Superior vena cava
Aorta — lg artery
pul. art.
pul. veins
Va veins
goes to lungs
R. atrium
R. ventricle
Inferior vena cava
Lower Body
pul. artery (to lungs)
pul. veins
left atrium
left ventricle
(muscle of the heart) myocardium muscle
Epicardium outer cov.

RA LA
RV LV

EXERCISE 18-4

Objective: To recognize and be able to correctly spell the names of various parts of the system of arteries.

Directions: Label the diagram in Figure 18-3 with the correct words from the word list below.

Word List

right common carotid	innominate artery	aortic arch
pulmonary artery	right subclavian artery	common iliac
descending aorta	left subclavian artery	femoral artery
left common carotid	right and left coronary arteries	ascending aorta

FIGURE 18-3

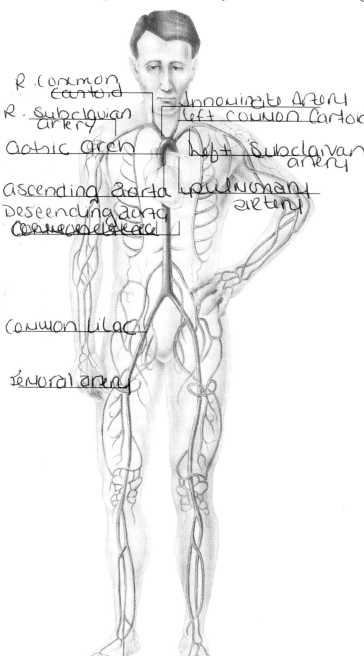

EXERCISE 18-5

Objective: To recognize and be able to correctly spell the names of various parts of the system of veins.

Directions: Label the diagram in Figure 18-4 with the correct words from the word list below.

Word List

internal jugular vein   external jugular vein   femoral vein
iliac vein   inferior vena cava   innominate vein
subclavian vein   superior vena cava

FIGURE 18-4

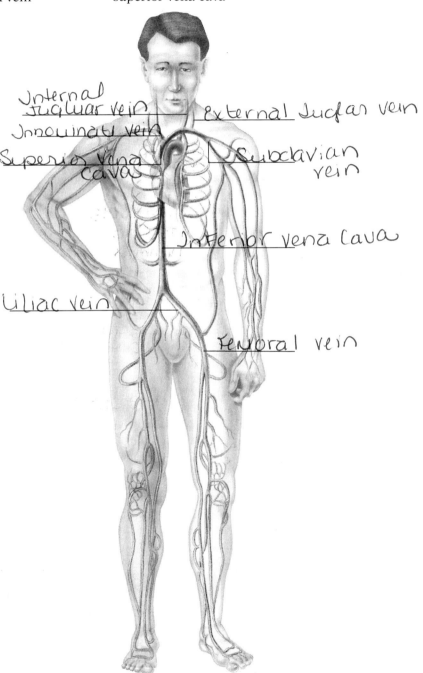

Internal Jugluar vein

Innouinatu vein

Superior vena cavas

external Juglar vein

Subclavian vein

Inferior vena Cava

Liliac vein

Femoral vein

EXERCISE 18-6

Objective: To recognize and be able to correctly spell the names of various parts of the respiratory system.

Directions: Label the diagram in Figure 18-5 with the correct words from the word list below.

Word List

adenoids	epiglottis	pleura	diaphragm
cells	ribs	tongue	pharynx
pulmonary artery	bronchiole	frontal sinus	tonsils
left main bronchus	pleural space	trachea	esophagus
pulmonary vein	alveolus (air sac)	capillaries	nasal cavity
bronchial cilia	oral cavity	mucus	
right main bronchus	larynx		

FIGURE 18-5

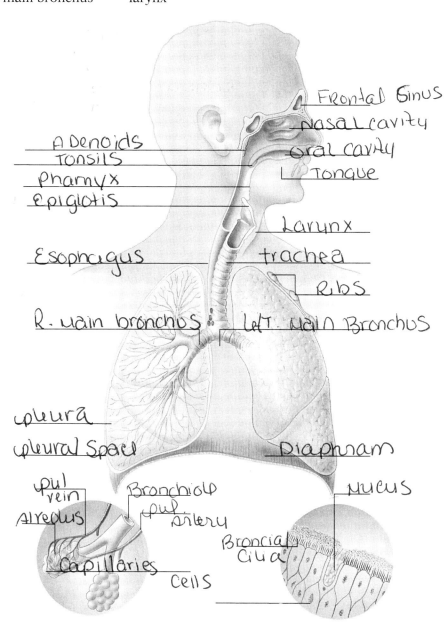

EXERCISE 18-7

Objective: To apply what you have learned about the circulatory system and related care.

Directions: Circle the letter next to the word or statement that best completes the sentence or describes the sentence as true or false. If the sentence is false, draw a line through the incorrect part of the sentence and write the correction on the blank line.

1. The _____ blood cells fight infection.
   A. red
   B. white
   C. plasma
   D. new
2. The heart is located in the chest cavity,
   A. pointing slightly to the patient's left.
   B. hanging low in the abdomen.
   C. pointing slightly to the patient's right.
   D. behind the large intestine.
3. The heart muscle must be supplied with blood
   A. carrying carbon dioxide.
   B. carrying oxygen.
   C. that is thick and slow.
   D. once every hour.
4. A pulmonary embolism is a blood clot that lodges in the
   A. feet.
   B. heart.
   C. brain.
   D. lungs.
5. A pulmonary embolism causes chest pain, difficulty in breathing, and
   A. is not serious.
   B. is treated with bed rest.
   C. is life-threatening.
   D. all of the above.
6. One reason older adults tire easily is that
   A. they are lazy.
   B. they do not get enough sleep.
   C. the brain has become smaller.
   D. the heart has reduced output because of weaker heart muscle.
7. The respiratory system makes it possible for
   A. urine to leave the blood.
   B. oxygen to move from the air into the blood.
   C. urine to enter the kidneys.
   D. blood to enter the brain.

8. Because we need oxygen to live, it is necessary to keep the respiratory system pathway (trachea, larynx, bronchi, lungs) open and functioning.
   A. True
   B. False
   Correct Answer: _____

9. If the epiglottis is not functioning, then _____ may occur.
   A. stomatitis
   B. epiglottitis
   C. aspiration into the lungs
   D. hypertension

10. In the lungs, the oxygen molecules get exchanged for carbon dioxide in the alveolar sacs.
    A. True
    B. False
    Correct Answer: _____exchanged____ w/ oxygen____

11. Chronic obstructive pulmonary disease (COPD) refers to a group of respiratory disorders, including all of the following except
    A. asthma.
    B. bronchitis.
    C. emphysema.
    D. tuberculosis.

12. The incidence of tuberculosis (TB) has been decreasing in recent years.
    A. True
    B. False
    Correct Answer: _____increasing_____

13. A patient with COPD will have difficulty
    A. swimming
    B. running.
    C. breathing.
    D. all of the above.

14. A person with obstructed breathing may mouth-breath and require
    A. more frequent mouth care.
    B. more back rubs.
    C. more steaming showers.
    D. more sleep.

15. Oxygen and carbon dioxide are also exchanged at the cellular level.
    A. True
    B. False
    Correct Answer: _____

16. The circulatory and respiratory systems
    A. are separate, and one is not affected by the other.
    B. are the same system.
    C. can take the place of the endocrine system.
    D. work closely together, and a condition that affects one may affect the other.

17. Patients who have diseases or limiting conditions of the circulatory or respiratory system will often find the activities of daily living difficult.
    A. True
    B. False
    Correct Answer: _____

18. After surgery, patients are encouraged to cough and deep-breathe to
    A. give them exercise.
    B. keep them oriented.
    C. expand the alveolar sacs and promote the exchange of oxygen.
    D. improve their coughing skills.

MEASURING VITAL SIGNS

The following exercises will assist you to apply what you have read in Chapter 19, "Measuring Vital Signs." For each exercise, read the objective and use information you have read in Chapter 19 to answer the questions, complete the sentences, or label the diagrams.

EXERCISE 19-1

Objective: To recognize the names of equipment commonly used to measure vital signs.

Directions: Label the pictures in Figure 19-1 with the number of the correctly matching name from the Word List below.

Word List

1. electronic oral/rectal thermometer
2. glass thermometer
3. disposable thermometer
4. aneroid sphygmomanometer
5. mercury sphygmomanometer
6. bell stethoscope
7. electronic ear thermometer
8. diaphragm stethoscope

FIGURE 19-1

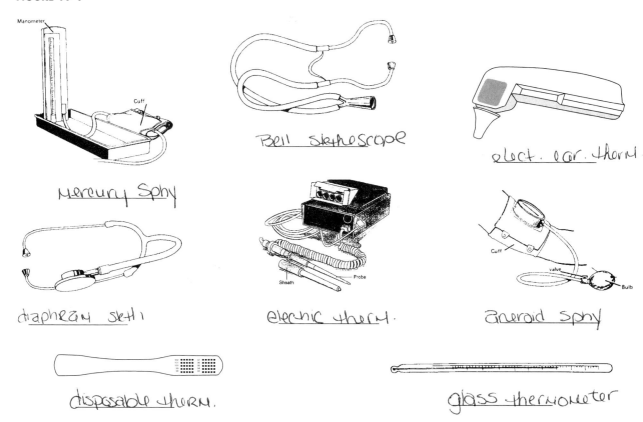

Mercury Sphy

Bell stethoscope

elect. ear. therm.

diaphram setti

electric therm.

aneroid sphy

disposable therm.

glass thermometer

EXERCISE 19-2

Objective: To recognize the definitions of words related to measuring vital signs.

Directions: Place the letter of the correct definition next to the matching word from the Word List.

Word List	Definitions
_N_ 1. labored respiration	A. The process of breathing out air in respiration
_O_ 2. mercury sphygmomanometer	B. A system for measuring temperature; in the Fahrenheit system, the temperature of water at boiling is 212°; at freezing, it is 32°; these temperatures are usually written 212°F and 32°F
_P_ 3. oral	C. Strength or power; used to describe the beat of the pulse
_Q_ 4. pulse	D. The process of breathing in air in respiration
_AA_ 5. systolic blood pressure	E. The depth of breathing changes and the rate of the rise and fall of the chest is not steady
_BB_ 6. thermometer	F. Breathing in which the patient is using mostly the abdominal muscles

Contracts

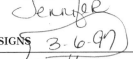

F   7. abdominal respiration

G   8. aneroid sphygmomanometer

Y   9. stertorous respiration

 10. stethoscope

K   11. centigrade

U   12. rectal

V   13. rhythm

H   14. apical pulse

I   15. axillary

J   16. blood pressure

L   17. Cheyne-Stokes respiration

R   18. pulse deficit

E   19. irregular respiration

S   20. radial pulse

T   21. rate

W   22. shallow respiration

23. sphygmomanometer

It's the Difrence in Between per minute

G. Dial-type blood pressure equipment

H. A measurement of the heartbeats at the apex of the heart, located just under the left breast

I. The area under the arms; the armpits

J. The force of the blood exerted on the inner walls of the arteries, veins, and chambers of the heart as it flows or circulates through the structure

K. A system for measurement of temperature using a scale divided into 100 units or degrees; in this system, the freezing temperature of water is 0°C and water boils at 100°C; often referred to as Celsius

L. One kind of irregular breathing. At first the breathing is slow and shallow; then the respiration becomes faster and deeper until it reaches a peak. The respiration then slows down and becomes shallow again. The breathing may then stop completely for 10 seconds and then begin the pattern again; this type of respiration may be caused by certain cerebral (brain), cardiac (heart), or pulmonary (lung) diseases or conditions

M. In taking a patient's blood pressure, one records the bottom number as the reading for the diastolic pressure; this is the relaxing phase of the heartbeat

N. Working hard to breathe

O. Blood pressure equipment containing a column of mercury

P. Anything to do with the mouth; examples are eating and speaking

Q. The rhythmic expansion and contraction of the arteries caused by the beating of the heart; the expansion and contraction show how fast, how regular, and with what force the heart is beating

R. A difference between the apical heartbeat and the radial pulse rate

S. This is the pulse felt at a person's wrist at the radial artery

T. Used to describe the number of pulse beats per minute

U. Pertaining to the rectum

V. Used to describe the regularity of the pulse beats

W. Breathing with only the upper part of the lungs

D 24. exhaling

auscultation

B 25. Fahrenheit

M 26. diastolic blood pressure

CC 27. apnea *no breathing*

C 28. force

A 29. inhaling

Dyspnea → Difficulty Breathing

X. An apparatus for measuring blood pressure

Y. The patient makes abnormal noises like snoring sounds when breathing

Z. An instrument that allows one to listen to various sounds in the patient's body, such as the heartbeat or breathing sounds

AA. The force with which blood is pumped when the heart muscle is contracting; when taking a patient's blood pressure, the systolic blood pressure is recorded as the top number

BB. An instrument used for measuring temperature

CC. Periods of not breathing

EXERCISE 19-3

Objective: To identify the common areas of the body where a pulse can be measured.

Directions: Label the diagram in Figure 19-2 with the correct word from the Word List below.

Word List

femoral pulse	temporal pulse	apical pulse	popliteal pulse
radial pulse	brachial pulse	pedal pulse	carotid pulse

FIGURE 19-2

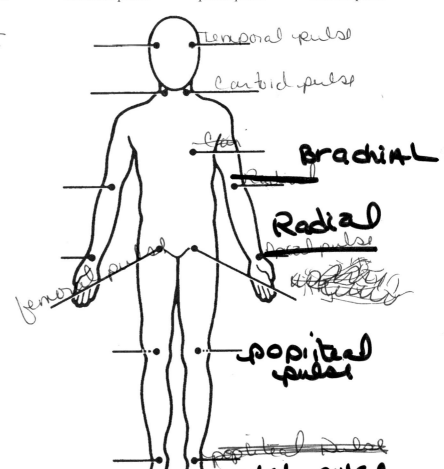

EXERCISE 19-4

Objective: To identify the correct technique for feeling the radial pulse.

Directions: Circle the letter next to the picture in Figure 19-3 that shows the correct technique for feeling the radial pulse.

FIGURE 19-3

A)

B)

C)

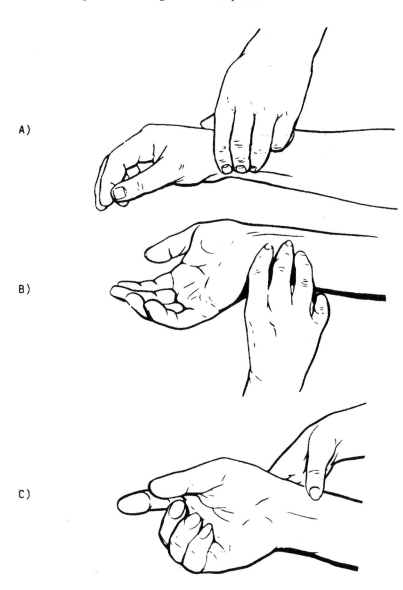

EXERCISE 19-5

Objective: To recognize important aspects of procedures used to measure vital signs.

Directions: Select from the List of Procedures the letter of the procedure that best answers each question. Write the correct letter(s) on the blank line(s) next to the question.

List of Procedures

A. Shaking down the glass thermometer
B. Reading a Fahrenheit thermometer
C. Reading a centigrade thermometer
D. Measuring an oral temperature
E. Measuring a rectal temperature
F. Measuring axillary temperature
G. Using a battery-operated electronic oral thermometer
H. Using a battery-operated electronic rectal thermometer
I. Using a battery-operated electronic oral thermometer to measure axillary temperature
J. Measuring the radial pulse
K. Measuring the apical pulse
L. Measuring the apical pulse deficit
M. Measuring respirations
N. Measuring blood pressure

1. Which procedure requires the use of a sphygmomanometer? _____
2. Which six procedures require the use of glass thermometers?

   _____   _____

   _____   _____

   _____   _____

3. Which two procedures could be used to get a measurement of R-100.4°F?

   _____ _____

4. In which three procedures would you observe the rate, rhythm, and force?

   _____ _____ _____

5. Which three procedures involve the use of a stethoscope? _____ _____

   _____

6. For which procedure would the normal adult rate be from 16 to 20 times a minute? _____

7. Which procedure could involve two nursing assistants working together?

   _____

8. Which procedure involves counting by twos like this: 2, 4, 6, 8? _____

9. Which three procedures would you follow if your immediate supervisor asked you to take vital signs? _____ _____ _____

10. Which two procedures could you use to measure temperature if the patient is receiving oxygen by cannula, catheter, face mask, or oxygen tent? _____

    _____

EXERCISE 19-6

Objective: To recognize important aspects of abnormal respirations.

Directions: Select the letters of the abnormal respiration from the Word List that match the definitions below. Write the letter next to the matching description.

Word List

A. stertorous respiration
B. abdominal respiration
C. shallow respiration

D. irregular respiration
E. Cheyne-Stokes respiration

1. _____ Breathing with only the upper part of the lungs
2. _____ Using mostly abdominal muscles for breathing
3. _____ A pattern where the breathing is slow and shallow, then faster and deeper to peak, then slow and shallow again. The breathing may stop for 10 seconds before beginning the pattern again.
4. _____ Abnormal sounds like snoring while breathing
5. _____ The depth and rate are not steady

EXERCISE 19-7

Objective: To identify important techniques for measuring respirations.

Directions: Circle the letter of the phrase that best completes the sentence.

1. To be sure the patient will not know that you are watching his breathing, you should
    A. count respirations while taking his temperature.
    B. hold the patient's wrist just as if you were taking his pulse.
    C. distract him by talking about the weather.
2. What should you do if you cannot clearly see the chest rise and fall?
    A. Fold the patient's arm across his chest to feel his breathing as you hold his wrist.
    B. Place your hand on the upper part of the patient's chest to feel his breathing.
    C. Call the head nurse or team leader as this might be an emergency.
3. If you count the chest rising 15 times in one full minute, you would report
    A. 30 respirations per minute.
    B. 15 respirations per minute.
    C. 7 respirations per minute.
4. If you count nine respirations in 30 seconds, you would report
    A. 27 respirations per minute.
    B. 9 respirations per minute.
    C. 18 respirations per minute.

5. If you count 19 respirations in a full minute, you would report
   A. 19 respirations per minute.
   B. 38 respirations per minute.
   C. 9 respirations per minute.

EXERCISE 19-8

Objective: To apply what you have learned about measuring the blood pressure.

Directions: Circle the letter of the word or phrase that best completes the sentence.

1. You are measuring the force of the blood flowing through the arteries when you
   A. measure a patient's temperature.
   B. count a patient's respirations.
   C. measure a patient's blood pressure.
   D. count a patient's pulse.
   E. measure a patient's vital signs.
2. "mm" is the abbreviation for
   A. mercury.   D. cubic centimeters.
   B. centimeters.   E. systolic.
   C. millimeters.
3. "Hg" is the abbreviation for
   A. mercury.   D. oxygen.
   B. centimeters.   E. diastolic.
   C. millimeters.
4. When a patient's blood pressure is higher than the normal range for his age and condition, it is referred to as
   A. hypotension.   D. millimeters mercury.
   B. high blood pressure.   E. low blood pressure.
   C. diastolic pressure.
5. When a patient's blood pressure is lower than the normal range for his age and condition, it is referred to as
   A. hypertension.   D. millimeters mercury.
   B. high blood pressure.   E. low blood pressure.
   C. diastolic pressure.
6. High blood pressure is also called
   A. hypotension.   D. diastolic pressure.
   B. hypertension.   E. Cheyne-Stokes pressure.
   C. systolic pressure.
7. Low blood pressure is also called
   A. systolic pressure.   D. hypotension.
   B. diastolic pressure.   E. hypertension.
   C. irregular pressure.

8. When you use a mercury sphygmomanometer, you will be
   A. watching the level of a column of mercury on a measuring scale.
   B. watching a pointer on a dial.
   C. counting respirations.
   D. watching a digital display.
   E. recharging the batteries.

9. When you use the aneroid sphygmomanometer, you will be
   A. watching the level of a column of mercury on a measuring scale.
   B. watching a pointer on a dial.
   C. counting respirations.
   D. watching a digital display.
   E. recharging the batteries.

10. When taking a patient's blood pressure, which two things will you be doing at the same time?
    A. listening to how the brachial pulse sounds in the brachial artery in the patient's arm.
    B. pumping air into the cuff.
    C. watching an indicator (either a column of mercury or a dial) to take a reading.
    D. counting respirations.
    E. both A and C.

11. When recording blood pressure you should write it $\frac{120}{80}$ or $^{120}\!/_{80}$. The top number stands for the
    A. systolic pressure.
    B. diastolic pressure.
    C. mercury pressure.
    D. blood pressure.
    E. millimeters mercury.

12. The bottom number of a recorded blood pressure stands for the
    A. systolic pressure.
    B. diastolic pressure.
    C. mercury pressure.
    D. blood pressure.
    E. millimeters mercury.

EXERCISE 19-9

Objective: To demonstrate your ability to correctly read an aneroid and a mercury sphygmomanometer.

Directions: Read the gauges in Figure 19-4 and write the correct answer on the blank line next to each gauge.

FIGURE 19-4

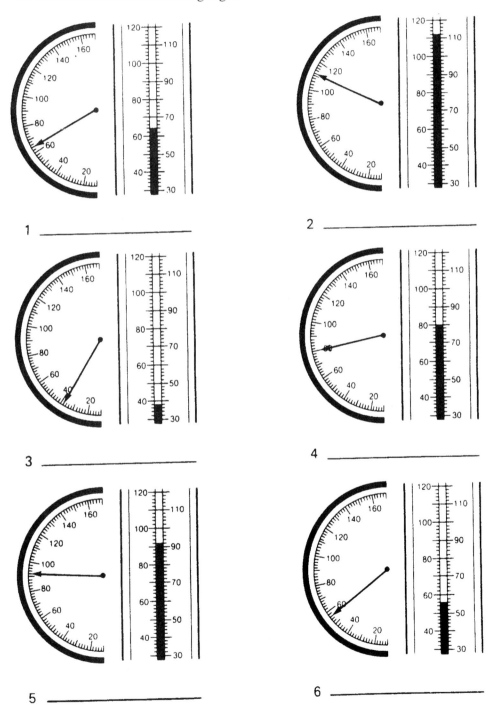

1 _____

2 _____

3 _____

4 _____

5 _____

6 _____

FIGURE 19-4 (cont.)

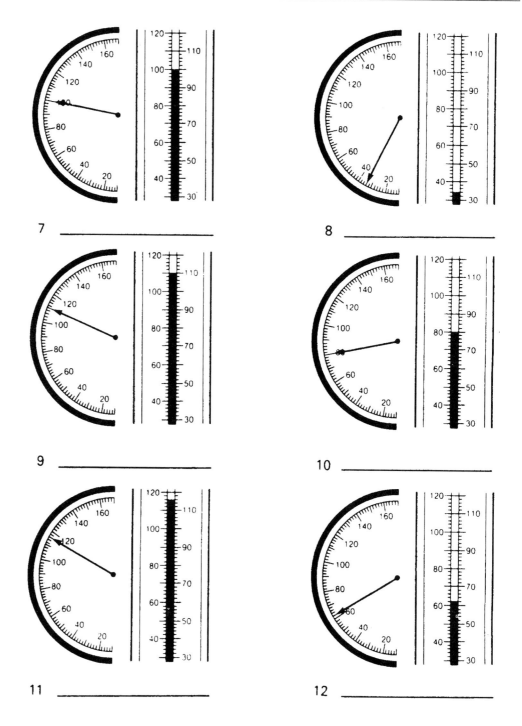

7 _____

8 _____

9 _____

10 _____

11 _____

12 _____

COMPETENCY CHECKLIST 19-1: VITAL SIGNS

ACTIVITY	S	U	COMMENTS
1. Student will correctly demonstrate the proper technique for:			
A. Shaking down a glass thermometer			
B. Reading a Fahrenheit thermometer			
C. Reading a centigrade thermometer			
D. Measuring an oral temperature			
E. Using a battery-operated electronic oral thermometer			
F. Measuring a rectal temperature using a glass thermometer			
G. Using a battery-operated electronic rectal thermometer			
H. Measuring an axillary temperature using a glass thermometer			
I. Using a battery-operated electronic oral thermometer to measure an axillary temperature			
J. Measuring a radial pulse			
K. Measuring an apical pulse			
L. Measuring an apical pulse deficit			
M. Measuring respiration			
N. Measuring blood pressure using a sphygmomanometer			

THE GASTROINTESTINAL SYSTEM AND RELATED CARE

The following exercises will assist you to apply what you have read in Chapter 20, "The Gastrointestinal System and Related Care." For each exercise, read the objective and use information you have read in Chapter 20 to answer the questions, complete the sentences, or label the diagrams.

EXERCISE 20-1

Objective: To recognize and correctly spell words related to the gastrointestinal system and related care.

Directions: Label the diagram in Figure 20-1 with the correct words from the Word List below.

Word List

mouth	teeth	tongue	salivary glands	liver
appendix	pancreas	stomach	pharynx	esophagus
large intestine	rectum	small intestine	gallbladder	duodenum

FIGURE 20-1   **THE GASTROINTESTINAL SYSTEM**

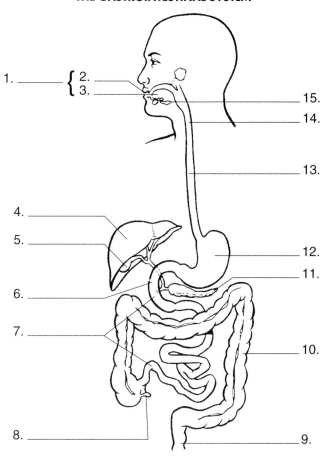

EXERCISE 20-2

Objective: To recognize and correctly spell words related to tube feedings and stomach lavage.

Directions: Label the diagram in Figure 20-2 with the correct words from the Word List below.

Word List

nostrils (naso)   esophagus   nasogastric feeding (gavage)
gastric irrigation (lavage) stomach (gastric)

FIGURE 20-2

GASTRIC GAVAGE AND LAVAGE

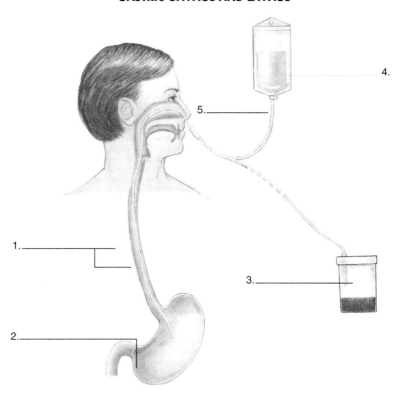

EXERCISE 20-3

Objective: To apply what you have learned about the gastrointestinal system and related care.

Directions: Read the following riddles carefully before writing the correct answer on the blank line.

1. These are 3 letters that stand for a certain kind of gastrostomy tube. What are the letters? *Hint:* An alternative meaning is something on which to hang your coat._____
2. These are 4 letters that stand for a certain kind of diet which is a remedy for diarrhea. What is it? *Hint:* An alternative meaning is the name for an unruly child._____
3. This word means a discharge of the lower bowel through the rectum and anus. What is it? *Hint:* An alternative meaning is something we do to remove people before or after a disaster strikes._____
4. This lubricating substance is put onto a rectal tube before insertion. What is it? *Hint:* It has been said that Santa Claus's stomach shakes like a bowlful of this._____

EXERCISE: 20-4

Objective: To recognize the definitions of words related to the gastro-intestinal system and related care.

Directions: Place the letter of the correct definition next to the matching word from the Word List.

Word List	Definitions
____ 1. gastrointestinal (GI) system	A. Discharge of the contents of the lower bowel through the rectum and anus
____ 2. suction	B. Procedure of evacuation or washing out of waste materials (feces or stool) from a person's lower bowel
____ 3. digestion	C. The first loop of the small intestine
____ 4. anus	D. Abnormally frequent discharge of fluid fecal material from the bowel
____ 5. absorption	E. Breaking down the food that is eaten into a form that can be used by the body cells
____ 6. small intestine	F. Uninterrupted, without a stop
____ 7. enema	G. Difficult, infrequent defecation, with passage of unduly hard and dry fecal material
____ 8. bile	H. Inflammation (swelling and irritation) of the appendix, typically with pain in the right lower quadrant
____ 9. Sims's position	I. The patient keeps the enema fluid (oil) in the rectum for 20 minutes
____ 10. lavage	J. Produces digestive juices and enzymes responsible for food breakdown in the small and large intestines
____ 11. gastrostomy tube (GT)	K. The secretion of the salivary glands into the mouth; contains an enzyme (protein) that helps digest starches
____ 12. flatus	L. An opening made through the abdomen to the stomach for the purpose of feeding
____ 13. retention	M. Feeding through a nasogastric tube
____ 14. diarrhea	N. Distal colon that absorbs water from stool
____ 15. constipation	O. Patient positioned on the left side with the right knee bent toward the chest, often called the enema position
____ 16. continuous	P. Using negative pressure to remove material, usually fluid
____ 17. rectum	Q. The GI tract is about 30 feet long and consists primarily of the mouth, esophagus, stomach, small intestine, and large intestine
____ 18. liver	R. The washing out of the stomach through a nasogastric tube, usually with normal saline
____ 19. pancreas	S. Muscular opening that controls elimination of stool from the rectum

____20. nasogastric tube

T. Part of the digestive process in which digestive juices and enzymes break down food into usable parts

____21. intermittent

U. The lowest portion of the large intestine, which curves in an *S*-shape and stores fecal material

____22. gastrostomy

V. Repeated washing out of the rectum. Clean water runs into the rectum, gas (flatus) and water run out of the rectum, as in the Harris flush.

____23. gavage

W. The first, smaller portion of the bowel, including the duodenum, where most of digestion and food breakdown occurs. Also known as the small bowel.

____24. peristalsis

X. Responsible for manufacturing bile and is a storage area for glucose. The liver also is the place where toxins, or poisons, are removed.

____25. duodenum

Y. A tube placed through one of the patient's nostrils (naso-), down the back of the throat, and through the esophagus into the patient's stomach (-gastric)

____26. rectal irrigation

Z. Rhythmic contractions of the muscle walls of the small and large intestines

____27. evacuation

AA. Alternating; stopping and beginning again

____28. appendicitis

BB. Tube inserted into the abdomen for the introduction of fluids

____29. large intestine

CC. Intestinal gas

____30. saliva

DD. Substance manufactured by the liver that helps the food breakdown process

EXERCISE 20-5

Objective: To apply what you have read about the gastrointestinal system and related care.

Directions: Circle the letter next to the word or statement that best completes the sentence or describes the sentence as true or false. If the sentence is false, draw a line through the incorrect part of the sentence and write the correction on the blank line.

1. Good nutrition and a functioning _____ are vital to a patient's health.
   A. nexus
   B. apex
   C. bowel
   D. tube

2. A large amount of _____ is necessary for the chemical breakdown of food.
   A. mercury
   B. lead
   C. water
   D. copper

3. The lining of the duodenum is composed of thousands of
    A. tilli.
    B. silli.
    C. billi.
    D. villi.

4. As a person ages, all of the following usually occur except
    A. the flow of saliva increases.
    B. the number of taste buds decreases.
    C. chewing and swallowing are more difficult.
    D. absorption of vitamins and minerals decreases.

5. All of the following are common disorders and diseases of the gastrointestinal system except
    A. myocardial infarction.
    B. hernias and ulcers.
    C. cholecystitis.
    D. constipation.

6. Varicose veins of the anal canal are called hemorrhoids.
    A. True
    B. False
    Correct Answer: _____

7. _____ are growths on the lining of the intestines that can become cancerous if not treated.
    A. Jauntoids
    B. Rectoids
    C. Polyps
    D. All of the above

8. When fluids are removed with a gravity nasogastric tube, it is important that the collecting container is higher than the patient's body.
    A. True
    B. False
    Correct Answer: _____

9. For removing fluids from a patient's body, the degree of suction most commonly used is
    A. high.
    B. low.
    C. intermittent.
    D. B and C.

10. Before giving fluid through the NG tube, listen with a stethoscope over the stomach while inserting air into the tube. The sound of air in the stomach means
    A. the tube is not properly placed.
    B. the lungs are inflating.
    C. the tube is loose.
    D. the tube is properly placed in the stomach.

11. If you notice that the formerly greenish fluid in the drainage container connected to the nasogastric tube has suddenly become bright red, what would you do?
    A. Empty the container when it is full.
    B. Measure and record the amount and color of the drainage.
    C. Notify your immediate supervisor at once.
    D. Tell the patient at once.

12. The nursing assistant is responsible for watching the level of the feeding and making sure the formula is being fed as fast as possible into the patient's stomach.
    A. True
    B. False
    Correct Answer: _____

13. In tube feeding, the formula is administered
    A. when thoroughly shaken and chilled.
    B. when it has reached boiling.
    C. at room temperature.
    D. at 98.6° F.

14. For adults, the NG tube must be flushed with 75 cc of water before and after the feeding or every eight hours.
    A. True
    B. False
    Correct Answer: _____

15. If the patient does not have a functioning GI tract, he may be able to receive a venous feeding called
    A. Total Parenteral Nutrition (TPN).
    B. Total Food Nutrition (TFN).
    C. Fast Food Nutrition (FFN).
    D. Venous Food Nutrition (VFN).

16. If a patient has diarrhea, it is important to also note the amount of _____ output, because it may indicate dehydration.
    A. blood
    B. work
    C. lavage
    D. urine

17. The most common cause of constipation is lack of adequate fluid intake.
    A. True
    B. False
    Correct Answer: _____

18. A device used to relieve flatus is
    A. high bulk foods.
    B. a rectal connector.
    C. a rectal tube with connected bag.
    D. a bowel bag.

19. Nursing assistants administer all of the following except
    A. a rectal tube.
    B. a medicated rectal suppository.
    C. a non-medicated rectal suppository.
    D. a back rub.

COMPETENCY CHECKLIST 20: GASTROINTESTINAL CARE

ACTIVITY	S	U	COMMENTS
1. The student will demonstrate the correct method of giving			
A. A cleansing enema			
B. The ready-to-use cleansing enema			
C. The ready-to-use oil retention enema			
D. the Harris Flush (return-flow enema)			
2. The student will demonstrate the correct method of using the disposable rectal tube with connected flatus bag.			
3. The student will demonstrate the correct method of administering a rectal suppository.			

NUTRITION FOR THE PATIENT

The following exercises will assist you to apply what you have read in Chapter 21, "Nutrition for the Patient." For each exercise, read the objective and use information you have read in Chapter 21 to answer the questions, complete the sentences, or label the diagrams.

EXERCISE 21-1

Objective: To recognize the definitions of words related to nutrition for the patient.

Directions: Place the letter of the correct definition next to the matching word from the Word List.

Word List	Definitions
____ 1. therapeutic diet	A. Counting or adding up a total of all calories consumed in a 24-hour period
____ 2. extra nourishment	B. Poor nutrition status
____ 3. nutrient	C. Delivery of a nutrition formula through a tube for patients with a functional GI tract who are unable to take in adequate calories or food by mouth
____ 4. enterally	D. Snacks
____ 5. omit	E. Any special diet
____ 6. nutrition status assessment	F. Nutrients needed for the human body to function; they must be consumed in the diet every day
____ 7. essential nutrients	G. Chemical substances found in foods
____ 8. malnutrition	H. Unit for measuring the energy produced when food is digested in the body
____ 9. calorie	I. Leave out
____ 10. registered dietitian (RD)	J. Nutrition therapy delivered by an IV catheter for patients with a nonfunctioning GI tract

____11. regular diet

    K. Assessment by an RN or RD as to what a patient eats and how the body uses it; determination of any special nutritional needs

____12. calorie count

    L. A basic, or well-balanced, diet containing appropriate amounts of foods from each of the food groups

____13. parenteral nutrition

    M. Person responsible for the preparation of well-balanced regular and therapeutic (special) diets to meet patients' nutritional needs

EXERCISE 21-2

Objective: To apply what you have learned about serving food to the patient.

Directions: More than one action may apply. Select the action that *most closely* addresses the situation. Write the letter of the correct action next to the matching situation below.

Actions

A. Check the tray yourself

B. Check the tray card against the ID band

C. Help any patient who needs it

D. Record this on appropriate form

E. Correct anything that is wrong or missing

Situations

____ 1. Before you give a tray to a patient

____ 2. To find the tray for each patient

____ 3. A patient cannot cut his meat

____ 4. A patient tells you he didn't get a fork

____ 5. The patient ate only half his food

____ 6. A patient tells you he has the wrong tray

____ 7. The patient refused to accept the tray and eats nothing

____ 8. Some food spills

____ 9. A patient seems too weak to pour his own coffee

____10. A patient on a regular diet didn't get any sugar on his tray, and he would like to have some

____11. You see a coffee pot on the patient's tray but no cup

____12. To be sure everything is on the tray

____13. A weak patient asks you to butter his bread

____14. The patient ate all the food served to him

____15. The patient tells you he didn't get any bread and butter, and you see none

EXERCISE 21-3

Objective: To apply what you have learned about passing drinking water to patients.

Directions: Write Do or Don't next to each statement below as appropriate.

1. _____ pass fresh drinking water to patients at the assigned intervals each shift or day.
2. _____ give ice to a patient whose pitcher is labeled "OMIT ICE".
3. _____ check to see which patients are NPO.
4. _____ check to see which patients are on restricted fluids.
5. _____ check to see which patients should get water *without ice*.
6. _____ return the same water pitcher to the patient from whom it was taken.
7. _____ remember to wash your hands before passing drinking water.
8. _____ wash your hands when done passing drinking water.

EXERCISE 21-4

Objective: To apply what you have learned about food groups.

Directions: Beside each food write the letter of the food group to which it belongs.

Food Groups

A. milk, yogurt, and cheese   B. vegetables   C. fruits

D. meat, poultry, fish, dried beans, eggs, and nuts   E. breads, cereals, rice, and pasta   F. fats, oil, sweets

Foods

_____ 1. peas
_____ 2. onions
_____ 3. milk
_____ 4. macaroni
_____ 5. broccoli
_____ 6. rice
_____ 7. bread
_____ 8. dried beans
_____ 9. yogurt
_____ 10. cake

_____ 11. nuts
_____ 12. carrots
_____ 13. potatoes
_____ 14. cheese
_____ 15. apple
_____ 16. butter
_____ 17. candy bar
_____ 18. blueberries
_____ 19. banana
_____ 20. chicken

EXERCISE 21-5

Objective: To apply what you have learned about essential nutrients.

Directions: For each food item listed below, find the nutrient that MOST CLOSELY matches that food item. Select each food item only once.

Nutrients

C = carbohydrates   P = protein   F = fat   W = water
V = vitamins   M = minerals

Foods

____ 1. margarine	____ 7. cheese
____ 2. beans	____ 8. meat
____ 3. beverages	____ 9. calcium
____ 4. fluoride	____10. biotin
____ 5. cereal	____11. iodine
____ 6. fruits	____12. butter

EXERCISE 21-6

Objective: To apply what you have learned about the most common types of diets.

Directions: For each diet type listed, read the common purpose and then fill in the description column. You may describe the diet and/or give examples.

Examples of Different Types of Patient Diets

TYPE OF DIET	DESCRIPTION	COMMON PURPOSE
1. Regular		To maintain or attain optimal nutritional status in patients who do not require a special diet.
2. Clear liquid		To provide calories and fluid in a form that requires minimal digestion. Commonly ordered after surgery.
3. Full liquid		For those unable to chew or swallow solid food. Used as a transitional diet between clear liquids and solid foods.
4. Soft		Used for patients who are unable to chew or swallow hard or coarse foods.
5. Mechanical soft		For patients with difficulty chewing or swallowing soft food.

TYPE OF DIET	DESCRIPTION	COMMON PURPOSE
6. Bland		Omits food that may cause excessive gastric acid secretion (ulcers).
7. Low residue		Used for patients with acute colitis, enteritis, and diverticulitis.
8. High residue/ fiber		Used for bowel regulation, high cholesterol, and high glucose; protects against colon cancer and diverticulosis.
9. Low calorie		For patients who need to lose weight.
10. Diabetic		For diabetic patients; matches food intake with the insulin requirements.
11. High protein		Assists in the repair of tissues wasted by disease. Used for increased protein needs (wound healing).
12. Low fat; low cholesterol		For patients who have difficulty digesting fat. Examples include patients with pancreatitis, cholestasis, heart and hepatic disease.
13. Lactose free/ low lactose		Used to prevent cramping and diarrhea in patients with a lactose deficiency.
14. Low sodium (low salt)		May be needed for patients with liver, cardiac, and renal disease. Used for patients with acute or chronic renal failure.
15. Gluten restricted		Used for patients with gluten sensitive enteropathy.

EXERCISE 21-7

Objective: To apply what you have learned about nutrition for patients.

Directions: Circle the letter next to the word or statement that best completes the sentence or describes the sentence as true or false. If the sentence is false, draw a line through the incorrect part of the sentence and write the correction on the blank line.

1. If you eat the recommended number of portions of foods from each food group on the pyramid every day, your diet will be
    A. adequate for body-builders.
    B. adequate for fast growth.
    C. adequate for good health.
    D. inadequate for patients.
2. The number and size of portions of food will depend on
    A. the age of the individual.
    B. the size of the individual.
    C. the activities of the individual.
    D. all of the above.
3. Calories from fat should be less than 60% of total calories.
    A. True
    B. False
    Correct Answer: _____
4. Fat has _____ calories per gram of fat.
    A. 100
    B. 9
    C. 4
    D. 90
5. Water has much caloric value.
    A. True
    B. False
    Correct Answer: _____
6. Alterations to the patient's diet may be necessary for all the following reasons except
    A. to increase or decrease the caloric content.
    B. a desire for fad dieting.
    C. to change the amounts of one or more nutrients.
    D. cultural or religious requirements.
7. The nutrition status assessment may include chewing or swallowing problems.
    A. True
    B. False
    Correct Answer: _____
8. Most patients would prefer
    A. to be fed.
    B. to feed themselves.
    C. to skip meals.
    D. to eat when nauseated.

COMPETENCY CHECKLIST 21: NUTRITION

ACTIVITY	S	U	COMMENTS
1. Student will demonstrate how to assist patients with foods:			
A. Preparing the patient for a meal			
B. Serving the food			
C. Feeding the physically challenged patient			
D. Serving the between-meal snack			
2. Student will demonstrate the correct method of passing drinking water.			

THE URINARY SYSTEM AND RELATED CARE

The following exercises will assist you to apply what you have read in Chapter 22, "The Urinary System and Related Care." For each exercise, read the objective and use information you have read in Chapter 22 to answer the questions, complete the sentences, or label the diagrams.

EXERCISE 22-1

Objective: To recall the correct definitions of words used in reference to the urinary system and related care.

Directions: Choose the correct word from the Word List and write it next to the appropriate definition.

Word List

fluid imbalance	force fluids	incontinent
calibrated	edema	urinary retention
fluid output	fluid intake	eliminate
urinary system	fluid balance	NPO
indwelling urinary catheter	void	homeostasis

Definitions

1. This word describes a measuring device marked with lines and numbers for measuring. _____

2. This term means to rid the body of waste products. _____

3. To voluntarily empty the bladder or urinate. _____

4. This term describes a patient who has a physician's order to not eat or drink, usually before surgery, a laboratory test, or a procedure or because his condition makes it necessary. _____

5. The group of body organs that includes the kidneys, ureters, bladder, and urethra. _____

6. The state of having stability of all body functions at normal levels. _____

7. When a patient is unable to voluntarily urinate, he is said to have a condition referred to as _____.

8. This is a tubular device that stays in the bladder and is used to drain out the urine. It often has a collection bag for the urine attached to it. _____ _____

9. This term describes a patient who is unable to control the excretion of feces or urine. _____

10. This situation can occur when either too much fluid stays in the body or too much fluid leaves the body. _____

11. The sum total of liquids that come out of the body. _____

12. _____ means that the amount of fluid eliminated is just about the same as the amount of fluid taken in.

13. The sum total of liquids that go into the body. _____

14. When the body retains excess fluid this condition can occur. _____

15. This order means that a patient is encouraged to drink fluids. _____ _____

EXERCISE 22-2

Objective: To recognize and be able to correctly spell the parts of the urinary system.

Directions: Label the diagram in Figure 22-1 with the correct words from the Word List below.

Word List

ureters	left kidney	bladder	nephron	Bowman's capsule
urethra	right kidney	glomerulus	tubule	

FIGURE 22-1

Organs of the Urinary System   Formation of Urine

EXERCISE 22-3

Objective: To correctly define words that refer to diseases and disorders of the urinary system.

Directions: Label each word with the letter of its correct definition.

Disease or Disorder		Definition
____ 1. Acute renal failure	A.	inflammation of the urinary bladder
____ 2. Anuria	B.	inflammation of the urethra often by sexually transmitted diseases such as chlamydia or gonorrhea.
____ 3. Cancer of the urinary bladder	C.	unusually large volume of urine in 24 hours
____ 4. Chronic renal failure	D.	painful voiding
____ 5. Cystitis	E.	frequency of urination at night
____ 6. Dysuria	F.	loss of kidney function
____ 7. Hematuria	G.	presence of pathogenic microorganisms in the urinary tract
____ 8. Hydronephrosis	H.	sharp, severe pain in lower back over kidney, accompany forcible dilation of a ureter due to a stone or urinary calculus
____ 9. Injury to the bladder	I.	presence of stones in the urinary (excretory) system
____10. Nocturia	J.	distention of the pelvis or one or both kidneys (urine being made but cannot be excreted due to urinary back up)
____11. Oliguria	K.	inability to urinate
____12. Polyuria	L.	very small amount of urine in 24 hours
____13. Pyeloneperitis	M.	caused by Myeobacterium tuberculosis in the kidney
____14. Pyuria	N.	pus in the urine infection
____15. Renal colic	O.	infection of the kidney (acute or chronic)
____16. Tuberculosis of the kidney	P.	malignant tumor
____17. Tumors of the kidney	Q.	no urine
____18. Urethral stricture	R.	narrowing of the urethra caused by infection or instrumentation; results in frequent voiding, dysuria, and hematuria (blood in the urine)
____19. Urethritis	S.	blood in the urine
____20. Urinary retention	T.	progressive deterioration of kidney function
____21. Urinary tract infection (UTI)	U.	considered malignant until proved otherwise
____22. Urolithiasis (renal calculi)	V.	due to trauma
____23. Dehydration	W.	Insufficient water in the tissues due to inadequate fluid intake or excessive fluid output

EXERCISE 22-4

Objective: To demonstrate the correct placement of intake and output information on the Intake and Output sheet.

Directions: Record the information in each statement in the correct place on the Intake and Output sheet in Figure 22-2. Total the amount for your shift. Refer to Figure 22-3 for the capacities of the serving containers.

PRACTICE STATEMENT: Mrs. Stavros is a patient who is dehydrated. She is on the Medicine Unit of the hospital where you are employed as a nursing assistant for the 7 A.M. to 3 P.M. shift. The doctor has ordered that she be put on a *liquid diet, force fluids* and that her fluid intake and output be measured for the next 24 hours. The nurse communicates to you in the morning report meeting that Mrs. Stavros will be your patient and that she will be on Intake and Output (I&O). The patient has not been taking fluids well, and so the nurse would like you to encourage her to increase her fluid intake. If her fluid intake does not improve in the next 24 hours, the doctor stated that she will order that an I.V. be started. She would prefer that the patient try to take her fluids orally if possible. Mrs. Stavros has an indwelling catheter.

Statements

1. Your patient drank one 6-oz cup of juice, drank one-half of a 12-oz bowl of broth, and ate one 6-oz Jell-O cup for breakfast.
2. Between breakfast and lunch, with your encouragement, she drank one 12-oz. can of ginger ale.
3. Your patient drank one 8-oz cup of milk, drank one-half of a 12-oz bowl of broth, and ate one 6-oz Jell-O cup for lunch.
4. Between lunch and the time your shift was over, you convinced her to drink one 8-oz cup of water.
5. When you measured the amount of urine in the catheter bag, you determined that it filled the graduate container to the one-quart level.

FIGURE 22-2

INTAKE				OUTPUT			
				URINE		GASTRIC	
ITEM	BY MOUTH	TUBE	PARENTERAL	VOIDED	CATHETER	EMESIS	SUCTION
TOTAL							

FIGURE 22-3

Examples of Capacities of Serving Containers

4-oz juice cup	120 cc
6-oz cup	180 cc
8-oz cup	240 cc
12-oz cup	360 cc
1-cup milk carton	240 cc
4-oz ice cream cup	120 cc
6-oz Jell-O cup	180 cc
6-oz coffee cup	180 cc
1-qt water pitcher	1000 cc

EXERCISE 22-5

Objective: To apply what you have learned about the urinary system and related patient care.

Directions: Circle the letter next to the word or statement that best completes the sentence or describes the sentence as true or false. If the sentence is false, draw a line through the incorrect part of the sentence and write the correction on the blank line.

1. Homeostasis is the body's attempt
   A. to keep its internal environment stable or in balance.
   B. to increase its fluid intake.
   C. to gain weight through fluid intake.
   D. to stand very still.
2. Diagnostic studies of the urinary system are
   A. body fat analyses and QID urinalyses.
   B. difficult to interpret.
   C. key to predicting growth rates in children.
   D. able to indicate kidney function.
3. Some body fluid is lost through
   A. perspiration.
   B. delegation.
   C. undulation.
   D. constipation.
4. An abbreviation for cubic centimeter is
   A. cb.ctr
   B. cc.
   C. cubo cento.
   D. cbcmtr.
5. The best time to record the patient's fluid intake is
   A. when you have time.
   B. when your immediate supervisor tells you to record ASAP.
   C. 20 minutes before the end of your shift.
   D. as soon as he consumes the fluids.
6. When measuring the capacity of serving containers, be sure to hold them at waist-level while carefully observing the amount of fluid.
   A. True
   B. False
   Correct Answer: _____
7. When measuring and recording intake and output, _____ _____ and _____ _____ are very important.
   A. good vision, good will
   B. exact observations, working fast
   C. disposable gloves, inline skates
   D. exact observations, accurate recordings

8. Fluids taken _____ are recorded by the nurse.
   A. intravenously
   B. secretly
   C. copiously
   D. daily
9. NPO means "note patient order".
   A. True
   B. False
   Correct Answer: _____
10. The indwelling catheter bag must always be kept
    A. above the head.
    B. above the waist.
    C. below the knee.
    D. below hip level.

COMPETENCY CHECKLIST 22-1: URINARY SYSTEM RELATED CARE

ACTIVITY	S	U	COMMENTS
1. Student correctly demonstrates measuring of serving containers.			
2. Student correctly demonstrates determining amounts consumed.			
3. Student correctly demonstrates measuring urinary output.			
4. Student correctly demonstrates emptying urine from an indwelling catheter container.			
5. Student correctly demonstrates giving daily indwelling catheter care.			

SPECIMEN COLLECTION

The following exercises will assist you to apply what you have read in Chapter 23, "Specimen Collection." For each exercise, read the objective and use information you have read in Chapter 23 to answer the questions, complete the sentences, or label the diagrams.

EXERCISE 23-1

Objective: To recognize the definitions of words related to specimen collection.

Directions: Place the letter of the correct definition next to the matching word from the Word List.

Word List	Definitions
____ 1. asepsis	A. Waste material coughed up from the lungs or trachea
____ 2. medical asepsis	B. A sample of material taken from the patient's body; examples are urine, feces, and sputum specimens
____ 3. saliva	C. Solid waste material discharged from the body through the rectum and anus; other names include excreta, excrement, bowel movement, and fecal matter
____ 4. expectorate	D. Catching the urine specimen between the time the patient begins to void and the time he stops
____ 5. clean catch	E. Special practices and procedures for preventing the conditions that allow disease-producing bacteria to live, multiply, and spread
____ 6. genital	F. Free of disease-causing organisms
____ 7. specimen	G. The secretion of the salivary glands into the mouth; saliva moistens food and helps in swallowing; it also contains an enzyme (protein) that helps digest starches

_____ 8. feces, stool

H. Refers to the fact that the urine for this specimen is not contaminated by anything outside the patient's body

_____ 9. midstream

I. To cough up matter from the lungs, trachea, or bronchial tubes and spit it out

_____ 10. sputum

J. Refers to the external reproductive organs

EXERCISE 23-2

Objective: To apply what you have learned about specimen collection.

Directions: Read the following carefully before writing the correct answer on the blank line.

1. This process is done to urine samples to detect solids in the urine. What is it? _____
2. This word describes a clean-catch urine specimen. What is it? _____
3. Feces is placed on this item when collected. What is it? _____
4. These can be found when the urine is strained. What are they? _____
5. When collecting a specimen, this item must be filled out with the proper information and sent to the laboratory with the specimen. What is it? _____

EXERCISE 23-3

Objective: To apply what you have learned about specimen collection.

Directions: Circle the letter next to the word or statement that best completes the sentence or describes the sentence as true or false. If the sentence is false, draw a line through the incorrect part of the sentence and write the correction on the blank line.

1. Most of the body's waste materials are discharged in the
    A. blood and sputum.
    B. sweat and mucus.
    C. urine and feces.
    D. stool and emesis.
2. If a person is sick, there will be noticeable changes in the body wastes when they are tested.
    A. True
    B. False
    Correct Answer: _____
3. Specimens are to be collected
    A. within 30 minutes of the ordered collection time.
    B. when the nursing assistant or nurse has time.
    C. at the exact time that is indicated.
    D. "whenever."

4. The specimen collection procedure must be followed exactly
    A. or the specimen may not be useful.
    B. in a step-by-step process.
    C. each time the specimen is collected.
    D. all of the above

5. It is very important to identify the patient by name, ID number, and room number before obtaining the specimen.
    A. True
    B. False
    Correct Answer: _____

6. The specimen must be _____ immediately to avoid mistakes.
    A. tested
    B. labeled
    C. stored
    D. shaken

7. If the specimen has the wrong name on it, all the following may occur except
    A. the wrong treatment may be ordered.
    B. the wrong medication may be ordered.
    C. the wrong problem may be identified.
    D. the patient will receive effective treatment.

8. It is important to wash your hands before and after collecting a specimen to avoid
    A. contamination of the specimen with your bacteria.
    B. spreading disease to the patient.
    C. contaminating yourself with disease-producing bacteria.
    D. all of the above

9. The urine specimen that is the most common is the
    A. routine urine specimen.
    B. fecal specimen.
    C. the common specimen.
    D. the institutional specimen.

10. A clean-catch specimen must be free from
    A. contamination.
    B. harm.
    C. cost.
    D. high temperatures.

11. A clean-catch specimen procedure requires careful washing of the abdominal area.
    A. True
    B. False
    Correct Answer: _____

12. Before a 24-hour urine specimen is started, the patient must
    A. shower for 24 minutes.
    B. be NPO for 24 hours.
    C. empty his bladder.
    D. measure his weight.

13. The last time the patient voids a sample to be included in the 24-hour specimen is
    A. exactly 24 hours after the start of the test.
    B. two days later.
    C. 24 hours after discharge.
    D. when 4 liters have been recorded.

14. Sputum is a substance collected from the patient's
    A. axilla.
    B. navel.
    C. sputola structures.
    D. lungs.

15. The best time to obtain a sputum specimen is in the early morning after the patient has been sleeping all night.
    A. True
    B. False
    Correct Answer: _____

16. The most common reason to test stool is to look for the presence of
    A. blood or parasites.
    B. stones or calculi.
    C. *E-coli* bacteria.
    D. bile.

17. Some stool specimens must be kept cold until tested.
    A. True
    B. False
    Correct Answer: _____

18. It is important to explain to the patient
    A. the reason for the test.
    B. the results of the test.
    C. what you are going to do before you do it.
    D. all the steps to be followed in collecting specimens.

COMPETENCY CHECKLIST 23: SPECIMEN COLLECTION

ACTIVITY	S	U	COMMENTS
1. Student will demonstrate the correct method for collecting urine specimens:			
A. Routine urine			
B. Infant routine urine			
C. Midstream clean-catch urine			
D. 24-hour urine			
2. Student will demonstrate the correct method for straining urine.			
3. Student will demonstrate the correct method for collecting a sputum specimen.			
4. Student will demonstrate the correct method for collecting a stool specimen.			
5. Student will demonstrate the correct method for preparing a hemoccult slide for feces testing.			

THE ENDOCRINE SYSTEM AND RELATED CARE OF DIABETICS

The following exercises will assist you to apply what you have read in Chapter 24, "The Endocrine System and Related Care of Diabetics." For each example, read the objective and use information you have read in Chapter 24 to answer the questions, complete the sentences, or label the diagrams.

EXERCISE 24-1

Objective: To recognize and correctly spell words related to the endocrine system and related care.

Directions: Label the diagram in Figure 24-1 with the correct words from the Word List below.

Word List

pineal	pituitary	parathyroids	testes (in men)	pancreas
thymus	thyroid	adrenals	ovaries (in women)	

FIGURE 24-1

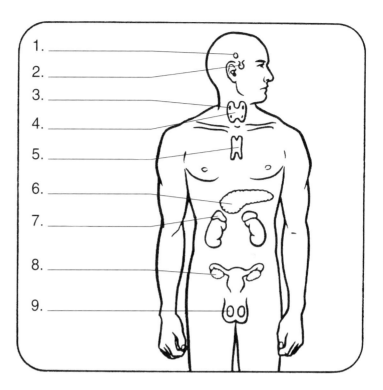

EXERCISE 24-2

Objective: To apply what you have learned about the endocrine system and related care of the diabetic.

Directions: Read the following riddles carefully before writing the correct answer on the blank line.

1. These are three classic symptoms of diabetes. What are they? *Hint:* The beginnings of all three words are the same and sound like a girl's name.

    _____

2. This item sounds like something you would write with, but it contains a point much sharper than a pen. What is it? *Hint:* It contains a lancet.

    _____

EXERCISE 24-3

Objective: To recognize the definitions of words related to the endocrine system and related care of the diabetic.

Directions: Place the letter of the correct definition next to the matching word from the Word List.

Word List	Definitions
____ 1. carbohydrate	A. A sugar formed during metabolism of carbohydrates; blood sugar.
____ 2. exocrine glands	B. To produce a special substance and release it.
____ 3. endocrine system	C. The process through which food substances are broken down in the body to yield energy.
____ 4. endocrine glands	D. Serious complication related to diabetes; occurs when the diabetic patient receives too much insulin, misses a meal, or has too much physical activity.
____ 5. hyperglycemia	E. A hormone produced naturally by the pancreas that helps the body change sugar into energy.
____ 6. insulin shock	F. Protein substances secreted by endocrine glands directly into the blood to stimulate increased activity.
____ 7. diabetes mellitus	G. Abnormally low blood sugar.
____ 8. metabolism	H. System composed of endocrine glands; regulates body function by secreting hormones.
____ 9. gland	I. Type of basic food element used by the body; composed of carbon, hydrogen, and oxygen; includes sugars and starches.
____ 10. hypoglycemia	J. Disorder of carbohydrate metabolism caused by inability to convert sugar into energy because of inadequate production or utilization of insulin.
____ 11. hormones	K. Glands that produce hormones and secrete them either directly or through a duct to epithelial tissue, such as a body cavity or the skin surface.
____ 12. glucose	L. An organ that is able to manufacture and discharge a chemical that will be used elsewhere in the body.
____ 13. insulin	M. Ductless glands that produce hormones and secrete them directly into the blood or lymph.
____ 14. secrete	N. Abnormally high blood sugar.
____ 15. diabetic coma	O. A coma (abnormal deep stupor) that can occur in a diabetic patient from lack of insulin.

EXERCISE 24-4

Objective: To apply what you have learned about the endocrine system and related care of the diabetic.

Directions: Circle the letter next to the word or statement that best completes the sentence or describes the sentence as true or false. If the sentence is false, draw a line through the incorrect part of the sentence and write the correction on the blank line.

1. The master gland of the body is the _____ gland.
    A. adrenal
    B. thyroid
    C. captain
    D. pituitary

2. The gland that is thought to be the link between our thinking, our emotions, and our body functions is the
    A. thinking link gland.
    B. hypothalamus gland.
    C. hippopotamus gland.
    D. emoto-gland.

3. Insulin is produced in the _____
    A. hypoinsulin gland.
    B. sugar gland.
    C. parathyroids.
    D. pancreas.

4. The thymus gland gets larger after puberty.
    A. True
    B. False
    Correct Answer: _____

5. In an emergency, the adrenal glands produce _____, which gives the body large amounts of energy.
    A. sugar
    B. insulin
    C. adrenalin
    D. progesterone

6. The adrenal glands lie on top of the
    A. throat.
    B. stomach.
    C. feet.
    D. kidneys.

7. Two female hormones are _____ and _____
    A. insulin, protectin.
    B. estrogen, testosterone.
    C. testosterone, insulin.
    D. estrogen, progesterone.

8. The _____ produces a hormone that regulates growth.
   A. pancreas
   B. thyroid
   C. heart
   D. stomach

9. Female hormones are produced in the
   A. ovaries.
   B. testes.
   C. pancreas.
   D. liver.

10. Male hormones are produced in the
    A. ovaries.
    B. testes.
    C. pancreas.
    D. liver.

11. Diabetes is a disease of the
    A. metabolism.
    B. nervous system.
    C. integumentary system.
    D. skeletal system.

12. _____ is a male hormone.
    A. Estrogen
    B. Progesterone
    C. Testosterone
    D. Insulin

13. Cushing's syndrome occurs when the adrenal glands are
    A. not active.
    B. too active.
    C. reactive.
    D. absent.

14. The most common disorder caused by endocrine problems is
    A. diabetes.
    B. obesity.
    C. pulmonary edema.
    D. Cushing's syndrome.

15. Gangrene can occur when a body part does not get enough
    A. insulin.
    B. circulating blood.
    C. gangrenite.
    D. pituitrin.

16. Signs and symptoms of diabetes include all of the following except
    A. polydipsia.
    B. polyphasia.
    C. polyuria.
    D. polyinsulin.

17. Symptoms of insulin shock include all of the following except
    A. faintness and dizziness.
    B. hyperglycemia.
    C. excessive sweating.
    D. irritability.
18. Signs of diabetic coma include all of the following except
    A. increased urination.
    B. loss of appetite.
    C. loss of consciousness.
    D. blurred vision.
19. _____ care is very important for diabetic health.
    A. Foot
    B. Hair
    C. Car
    D. Home
20. Good control of blood sugar levels is dependent upon use of _____ _____.
    A. foot meters.
    B. insulin meters.
    C. carbohydrate meters.
    D. blood glucose meters.
21. It is important that the patient learn to use a blood glucose meter and to administer his own insulin.
    A. True
    B. False
    Correct Answer: _____
22. For diabetics, shoes and stockings should fit correctly and not be
    A. too tight.
    B. too loose.
    C. constrictive.
    D. all of the above.
23. When using a blood glucose meter for several patients, the nursing assistant should
    A. use a pipet to prevent contamination of the patient.
    B. wash his hands between patients.
    C. be sure to record the blood level after each test.
    D. all of the above.
24. The nursing assistant must always wear disposable gloves when testing the patient's blood.
    A. True
    B. False
    Correct Answer: _____
25. Whenever testing the urine, use
    A. a fresh sample.
    B. a sample from the Foley bag.
    C. a sample from the last test.
    D. a sample from the toilet.

COMPETENCY CHECKLIST 24: GLUCOSE TESTING

ACTIVITY	S	U	COMMENTS
The student will demonstrate the correct method of testing for glucose using the One-Touch Profile diabetes tracking system.			

THE REPRODUCTIVE SYSTEM AND RELATED CARE

The following exercises will assist you to apply what you have read in Chapter 25, "The Reproductive System and Related Care." For each exercise, read the objective and use information you have read in Chapter 25 to answer the questions, complete the sentences, or label the diagrams.

EXERCISE 25-1

Objective: To recognize and be able to correctly spell the parts of the female reproductive system.

Directions: Label in Figure 25-1 the parts of the female reproductive organs and specialized cells with the words from the Word List.

Word List

labia majora	uterus
ovary tube	cervix
uterine neck	urethral meatus
fallopian tube	vaginal orifice
labia minora	hymen
ovary	clitoris
ovum escaping	vagina or birth canal

FIGURE 25-1

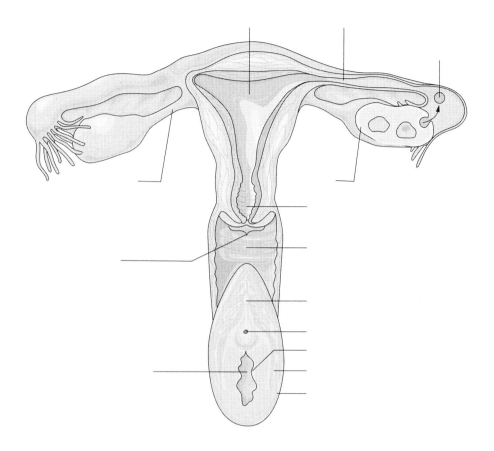

EXERCISE 25-2

Objective: To recognize and be able to correctly spell the parts of the male reproductive organs.

Directions: Label in Figure 25-2 the parts of the male reproductive organs and specialized cells with the words from the Word List.

Word List

bladder	testicle (testis)
glans penis	vas deferens
prostate	epididymis
bulbo-urethral gland	urethral meatus
rectum	prepuce
ejaculatory duct	scrotum
seminal vesicle	

FIGURE 25-2

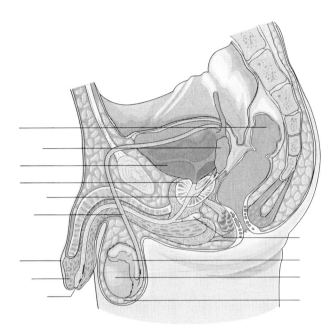

EXERCISE 25-3

Objective: To associate sexually transmitted diseases (STDs) with their responsible organisms.

Directions: Draw a line to connect the disease with the correct organism.

chlamydia	HPV virus
gonorrhea	herpes simplex virus
AIDS	Chlamydia
syphilis	gonococcus
genital herpes simplex	HIV virus
genital warts	*Treponema pallidum*

EXERCISE 25-4

Objective: To identify words that relate to postpartum care.

Directions: Unscramble the words in the Word List at the left. Then circle the same words in the Word Search grid at the right.

Word List

1. MUVO _____

2. TRAPTUMPOS _____

3. MERSP _____

4. XVIRCE_____

5. TINMOLAUAB_____

6. NEARCASE ECSTION_____

7. IPRE TOLBET_____

8. CAVRIPY_____

Word Search

O	Q	A	S	P	R	I	V	A	C	Y	X	W	U	P	X
V	Y	P	E	R	I	B	O	T	T	L	E	G	S	U	W
U	C	E	S	A	R	E	A	N	S	E	C	T	I	O	N
M	K	R	Q	A	M	B	U	L	A	T	I	O	N	Q	R
S	K	N	B	V	C	X	U	P	W	P	I	M	I	L	A
P	E	R	C	E	R	V	I	X	R	M	W	O	M	I	L
E	P	I	Q	P	O	S	T	P	A	R	T	U	M	K	F
R	C	V	E	T	Y	P	M	T	B	U	W	X	I	L	S
M	O	T	R	E	V	C	Q	R	T	X	W	E	E	N	C

EXERCISE 25-5

Objective: To recall important points to remember when preparing a female patient for a pelvic examination.

Directions: Complete the following sentences with the correct words from the Word List below. You are a nursing assistant who has been working for 6 months after completing your training. You work in a women's health clinic. The nurse asks you to prepare Ms. Smith for a pelvic exam.

1. This examination is very important for assessing the _____ of the female _____ organs.
2. This can be a difficult _____ for a woman to receive.
3. It is important that _____ and _____ be maintained.
4. The typical position used in this exam is the _____ position.
5. _____ may be used to position the legs and the feet.
6. An additional _____ may be used to cover the feet.
7. If you leave the patient alone in the room, make sure to leave the _____ _____ within her reach.
8. _____ your _____ before and after handling equipment or specimens and use disposable _____ .
9. Care for the _____ according to the clinic's policy.
10. After the examination, assist the patient to _____ or put on a _____ . If she is able to dress herself, leave the room so that the patient can dress herself in private.

EXERCISE 25-6

Objective: To apply what you have learned about human reproduction and patient care.

Directions: Circle the letter next to the statement that best completes the sentence or describes the sentence as true or false. If the sentence is false, draw a line through the incorrect portion of the sentence.

Word List

condition	gown	drape	call light	privacy
stirrups	wash	gloves	examination	comfort
equipment	dress	hands	dorsal lithotomy	reproductive

1. There are several female organs of reproduction, but the primary reproductive organs are the
   A. uterus and the vagina.
   B. two ovaries.
   C. fallopian tubes.
   D. testes and the penis.
2. The primary reproductive organs of the male are the
   A. two testes.
   B. penis and the prostate gland.
   C. sperm cells.
   D. urethra and the penis.
3. Estrogen and progesterone are male hormones.
   A. True
   B. False
   Correct Answer: _____
4. The process whereby an ovum is released from an ovary into the fallopian tubes and travels to the uterus is called
   A. inspiration.
   B. climax.
   C. menstruation.
   D. ovulation.
5. During intercourse, the sperm travel up the vas deferens to a point where they enter the urethra.
   A. True
   B. False
   Correct Answer: _____
6. Menstruation diminishes around age 45–52, leading to menopause.
   A. True
   B. False
   Correct Answer: _____

7. In the human female there are three openings in the perineal area; these are called the
   A. urethra, the cervix, and the penis.
   B. scrotum, the urethra, and the anus.
   C. vagina, the urethra, and the anus.
   D. vagina, the urethra, and the uterus.

8. There is only one duct in the penis that is used for the flow of urine and the flow of
   A. blood.
   B. milk.
   C. testosterone.
   D. semen.

9. Sexuality refers to the group of characteristics that identify the differences between
   A. sex and reproduction.
   B. good and bad.
   C. right and wrong.
   D. male and female.

10. Sexuality is a normal part of growth and development and must always be associated with the sex organs.
    A. True
    B. False
    Correct Answer: _____

_____

11. Sexually transmitted diseases (STDs) can be 100% prevented
    A. by luck and timing.
    B. through abstinence.
    C. by the use of male condoms.
    D. by the use of female condoms.

12. A person can carry the HIV virus for many years before developing AIDS.
    A. True
    B. False
    Correct Answer: _____

13. Three examples of STDs are
    A. Chlamydia, pneumonia, and gonorrhea.
    B. Chlamydia, gonorrhea, and amenorrhea.
    C. HSV, HPV, and HIV.

14. Genital herpes simplex (HSV) can be contracted
    A. only if sores are visable.
    B. only if sores are open and draining.
    C. from anyone having HSV.
    D. only during menstruation.

15. Some forms of human papillomavirus (HPV) infection (genital warts) can be cancerous.
    A. True
    B. False
    Correct Answer: _____

16. Examples of female reproductive disorders are
    A. cystocele and rectocele.
    B. tumors of the breast and hydrocele.
    C. prostatitis and BPH.
    D. varicocele and varicose veins.

17. Examples of male reproductive disorders are
    A. prostatitis and benign prostatic hyperplasia (BPH).
    B. tumors of the breast and cancer of the uterus.
    C. vaginitis and pelvic inflammatory disease (PID).
    D. menorrhagia and backaches.

18. Another word for vaginal irrigation is
    A. constipation.
    B. enema.
    C. douche.
    D. perineal care.

19. An episiotomy is a small cut in the vagina made during childbirth to make the opening larger and to prevent tearing.
    A. True
    B. False
    Correct Answer: _____

20. Postpartum perineal care is performed each time after the patient urinates and/or defecates.
    A. True
    B. False
    Correct Answer: _____

21. Postpartum perineal care differs from other perineal care for females because
    A. the patient performs this procedure only by herself.
    B. ice water must be used.
    C. a peri bottle filled with warm water is used.
    D. it can be performed only after eating.

22. A sleepy nursing mother may need
    A. a list of ten easy ways to stay awake.
    B. loud music played whenever nursing the baby.
    C. the siderails up for safety while feeding the baby.
    D. a cold shower before nursing the baby.

23. Early ambulation is important to prevent circulation problems after child-birth, but before the patient gets up you must check with your immediate supervisor to see if the patient
    A. has hardsole shoes to wear.
    B. has numbness in her legs from the anesthesia.
    C. has orders to walk more than a mile a day.
    D. can request that her husband walk for her.

24. Some patients develop a severe rash if they ambulate when they have doctor's orders to lay flat or at a reduced angle for several hours after receiving spinal anesthesia.
    A. True
    B. False
    Correct Answer: _____

25. The way a patient expects to be treated by a health care worker is influenced by
    A. the time of day.
    B. the nurse.
    C. pain.
    D. the cultural characteristics of that patient.

COMPETENCY CHECKLIST 25-1: CARE RELATED TO THE REPRODUCTIVE SYSTEM

ACTIVITY	S	U	COMMENTS
1. Student will demonstrate the proper procedure for preparing the female patient for a pelvic exam.			
2. Student will demonstrate the proper procedure for performing postpartum perineal care.			

THE NERVOUS SYSTEM AND RELATED CARE

The following exercises will assist you to apply what you have read in Chapter 26, "The Nervous System and Related Care." For each exercise, read the objective and use information you have read in Chapter 26 to answer the questions, complete the sentences, or label the diagrams.

EXERCISE 26-1

Objective: To recognize and correctly spell words related to the nervous system and related care.

Directions: Unscramble the words in the Word List at the left. Then circle the same words in the Word Search at the right.

Word List

1. BEMOLSU _Embolus_
2. ULESPMI _impulse_
3. QAEULP _plaque_
4. TRUPUER _Rupture_
5. UEZRESI _Seizure_
6. IHMPELGEAI _Hemiplegia_
7. FDECITI _deficit_
8. PASAHAI _Aphasia_

Word Search

K	I	L	C	T	D	E	B	A	G	R	F	N	Q
D	R	T	K	F	O	S	F	O	I	U	U	D	S
H	W	E	M	B	O	L	U	S	L	P	I	E	A
E	O	U	K	Q	E	U	R	M	D	T	M	F	S
L	P	A	N	A	G	P	L	A	Q	U	E	I	H
P	Q	I	D	H	S	M	C	L	A	R	L	C	I
L	M	S	A	B	F	I	I	B	J	E	C	I	S
R	G	A	F	I	C	F	S	A	E	F	B	T	P
V	L	H	S	E	I	Z	U	R	E	D	G	G	M
A	R	P	E	R	D	G	J	B	Q	K	A	H	O
I	P	A	I	G	E	L	P	I	M	E	H	K	V
X	I	C	P	A	H	M	T	J	S	B	O	L	W
A	E	U	K	Z	L	O	S	W	N	N	I	D	T

EXERCISE 26-2

Objective: To apply what you have learned about the nervous system and related care.

Directions: Read the following riddles carefully before writing the correct answer on the blank line.

1. I often form on the inside of vessel walls. Who am I? *Hint:* My name sounds like an engraved award. _Plaque_

2. When I occur, I can cause the patient to become unconscious. Who am I? *Hint:* Under different circumstances, I would take your possessions away.
    Seizure

EXERCISE 26-3

Objective: To recognize the definitions of words used in patient rehabilitation activities.

Directions: Place the letter of the correct definition next to the matching word from the Word List.

	Word List		Definitions
E	1. cerebral spinal fluid	A.	Excessive bleeding
M	2. intervertebral discs	B.	An area of the brain responsible for control of the pituitary gland
G	3. canthus	C.	The part of the nervous system that carries messages without conscious thought
F	4. aphasia	D.	An electrical or chemical charge transmitted through certain tissues, especially nerve fibers and muscles
A	5. hemorrhage	E.	The fluid that circulates around and within the brain and spinal cord
C	6. autonomic nervous system	F.	Loss of language or speech
DD	7. involuntary	G.	The inner aspect of the eye closest to the nose
D	8. embolus	H.	A seizure with motor and possible sensory symptoms (such as muscle twitching and smelling a foul odor) and a change in the level of consciousness
Q	9. contracture	I.	All the surrounding conditions and influences affecting the life and development of an organism
L	10. myelin sheath	J.	A temporary or permanent negative change in a patient's usual neurologic function
HH	11. cerebrovascular accident (CVA)	K.	Fatty deposits within blood vessels attached to vessel walls
R	12. rupture	L.	Protective covering around most nerves
BB	13. meninges	M.	The material between the vertebral bodies that cushions the spinal column

_B_ 14. hypothalamus

_I_ 15. environment

_I_ 16. convulsive

_Y_ 17. deficit

_H_ 18. complex partial seizure

_K_ 19. plaque

_X_ 20. osteoporosis

_GG_ 21. stimuli

_U_ 22. seizure

_EE_ 23. spasm

_II_ 24. simple partial seizure

_W_ 25. voluntary

_S_ 26. nervous system

_CC_ 27. hemiplegia

_FF_ 28. vascular

_D_ 29. impulse

_Y_ 30. neuron

_AA_ 31. thrombus

_V_ 32. vertebral bodies

_O_ 33. respond

_N_ 34. hemisphere

N. Half of a sphere; in the nervous system it refers to one-half of the brain

O. To react; to begin, end, or change activity in reaction to stimulation

P. A blood clot or mass of other undissolved matter that travels through the circulatory system from its place of formation to another site, lodges in a small blood vessel, and causes an obstruction

Q. When muscle tissue becomes drawn together, bunched up, or shortened because of spasm or paralysis, either permanently or temporarily

R. Break open

S. The group of body organs consisting of the brain, spinal cord, and nerves that controls and regulates the activities of the body and the functions of the other body systems

T. With convulsions present. Convulsions are rhythmic, involuntary contractions of muscles

U. An episode, either partial or generalized, that may include altered consciousness, motor activity, or sensory phenomena or convulsions

V. The bones of the spinal cord

W. Under control of the will

X. Condition in which bones become brittle or thin and break easily

Y. A type of nerve cell in the nervous system

AA. A blood clot that remains at its site of formation

BB. The covering of the brain and spinal cord. There are three layers: the dura mater, the arachnoid, and the pia mater

CC. Paralysis of only one-half of the body

DD. Without conscious will, control, or decision

EE. An involuntary sudden movement or convulsive muscular contraction

FF. Pertaining to blood vessels

GG. Changes in the external or internal environment strong enough to set up a nervous impulse or other responses in an organism

HH. Stroke; blood vessels in the brain become blocked or bleed, interrupting the blood supply to that part of the brain and damaging the surrounding area of the brain

II. A seizure when the patient is aware of his surroundings but experiences either motor (muscle twitching or movement) or sensory changes (see or hear things not present)

EXERCISE 26-4

Objective: To recognize the structures and functions of the nervous system.

Directions: Label the drawings in Figure 26-1 utilizing the words from the Word List below. (Some answers may be used more than once.)

Word List

cerebrum	cerebellum	brain	pons
spinal nerves	medulla	axon	neuron
nucleus	dendrite	motor neuron	muscle tissue
myelin sheath	sensory message to the brain		spinal cord*
motor message from the brain			

*This word is used twice in Figure 26-1.

FIGURE 26-1

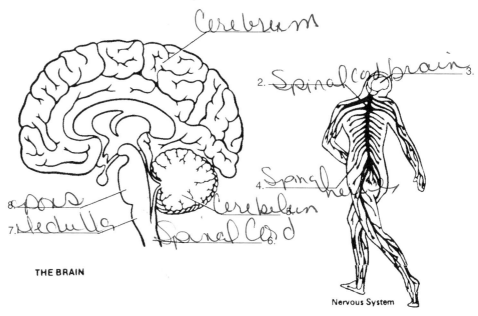

THE BRAIN

Nervous System

FIGURE 26-1 (cont)

SENSORY AND MOTOR PROCESSES IN OPERATION

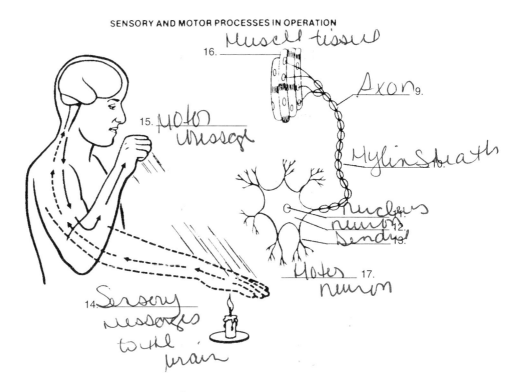

16. _Muscle tissue_

Axon 9.

15. _Motor message_

Mylin Sheath 10.

Nucleus neurons 12.

Dendrite 13.

17. _Motor neuron_

14. _Sensory messages to the brain_

EXERCISE 26-5

Objective: To apply what you have learned about the nervous system and related care.

Directions: Circle the letter next to the statement that best completes the sentence or describes the sentence as true or false. If the sentence is false, draw a line through the incorrect part of the sentence and write the correction on the blank line.

1. We are aware of our environment through our
    A. digestive organs.
    B. sense organs.
    C. response organs.
    D. all of the above.
2. For the patient who has an _____, cleaning it is part of daily personal hygiene.
    A. artificial eye
    B. imagination
    C. missing canthus
    D. old injury
3. A hearing aid will restore full, normal hearing ability.
    A. True
    B. False
    Correct Answer: _will not partial_

4. A hearing aid has all of the following except
   A. an amplifier.
   B. a telegram.
   C. an earmold.
   D. a microphone.

5. The weight and size of the brain decrease as a person ages.
   A. True
   B. False
   Correct Answer: _____

6. _____ is a weakness or paralysis of one side of the face.
   A. Bell's palsy
   B. Bob's bell
   C. Paul's bell
   D. Belle's pal

7. _____ may be related to cerebral trauma.
   A. Osteoporosis
   B. Alopecia
   C. Dermatitis
   D. Epilepsy

8. A disease that is a type of dementia is
   A. glaucoma.
   B. vertigo.
   C. Alzheimer's.
   D. a detached retina.

9. Blisters along the path of certain nerves is known as
   A. shingles (*Herpes zoster*).
   B. quadriplegia.
   C. cataracts.
   D. Meniere's disease.

10. Parkinson's disease is a progressive disorder, leading to loss of control of movement.
    A. True
    B. False
    Correct Answer: _____

COMPETENCY SKILLS CHECKLIST 26: NERVOUS SYSTEM CARE

ACTIVITY	S	U	COMMENTS
1. Student will demonstrate the proper method of caring for the artificial eye.			
2. Student will demonstrate the proper method of caring for the patient's eyeglasses.			
3. Student will demonstrate the proper method of applying the hearing aid.			

WARM AND COLD APPLICATIONS

The following exercises will assist you to apply what you have read in Chapter 27, "Warm and Cold Applications." For each exercise, read the objective and use information you have read in Chapter 27 to answer the questions, complete the sentences, or label the diagrams.

EXERCISE 27-1

Objective: To recognize and correctly spell words related to warm and cold applications.

Directions: Unscramble the words in the Word List at the left. Then circle the same words in the Word Search at the right.

Word List	Word Search

Word List

1. NOITAMMALFNI _____

2. CLAOLZIDE _____

3. OMSTI _____

4. OASK _____

5. MOCRSEPS _____

6. ETHA _____

7. CANYSOIS _____

8. DCLO _____

Word Search

C	G	B	L	S	O	A	S	E	F	C	N	K
B	H	E	A	T	V	I	L	D	F	O	C	L
V	D	I	K	J	S	C	F	G	I	M	B	X
F	R	P	A	O	Z	H	X	T	D	P	D	P
U	F	Q	N	R	D	G	A	Q	Y	R	H	O
L	X	A	K	O	A	M	L	A	B	E	C	H
H	Y	B	S	B	M	S	Y	M	C	S	O	Z
C	D	O	C	A	A	E	D	O	T	S	L	N
A	Z	J	L	O	C	A	L	I	Z	E	D	S
E	S	F	Y	I	D	V	L	S	F	A	L	Y
G	N	I	C	D	J	G	B	T	M	A	L	Z
I	A	F	B	S	O	A	K	H	K	B	C	J
K	H	N	L	P	V	O	W	S	T	X	O	W

EXERCISE 27-2

Objective: To apply what you have learned about warm and cold applications.

Directions: Read the following riddles carefully before writing the correct answer on the blank line.

1. I describe how something can get smaller or narrower. What am I? *Hint:* My alternate definition is legally binding. _____
2. This is a treatment that patients report as warm and soothing. What is it? *Hint:* To walk, a person is standing. To drive a car, he _____
3. This cold application can cool a warm head. What is it? *Hint:* There is also one of these at the North and South Poles. _____

EXERCISE 27-3

Objective: To recognize the definitions of words related to the use of warm and cold applications.

Directions: Place the letter of the correct definition next to the matching word from the Word List.

Word List	Definitions
____ 1. continuous	A. A bath in which the patient sits in a specially designed chairtub or a regular bathtub with the hips and buttocks in water
____ 2. dilate	B. Get bigger; expand
____ 3. localized application	C. A warm or cold application in which water touches the body
____ 4. cyanosis	D. Immerse the body or body part completely in water
____ 5. compress	E. Get smaller
____ 6. dry application	F. A warm or cold application applied to a specific area or small part of the body
____ 7. constrict	G. Alternating; stopping and beginning again
____ 8. soak	H. When the skin looks blue or gray, especially on the lips, nailbeds, and under the fingernails. In a black patient, it may appear as a darkening of color. This occurs when there is not enough oxygen in the blood
____ 9. generalized application	I. Uninterrupted, without a stop
____10. localized	J. Folded piece of cloth used to apply pressure, moisture, heat, cold, or medication to a specific part of the body
____11. sitz bath	K. A warm or dry application in which no water touches the skin
____12. moist application	L. Affecting, involving, or pertaining to the whole body

_____13. intermittent   M. Limited to one place or part; affecting, involving, or pertaining to a definite area

_____14. inflammation   N. A warm or cold application applied to the entire body

_____15. generalized   O. A reaction of the tissues to disease or injury; there is usually pain, heat, redness, and swelling of the body part

EXERCISE 27-4

Objective: To apply what you have learned about using warm and cold applications.

Directions: Circle the letter next to the statement that best completes the sentence or describes the sentence as true or false. If the sentence is false, draw a line through the incorrect part of the sentence and write the correction on the blank line.

1. Heat may be applied to an area of the body to
   A. improve the patient's appearance.
   B. improve the appearance of the skin.
   C. speed up the healing process by increasing the circulation.
   D. speed up the healing process by decreasing the circulation.

2. Heat may also be applied to the body to
   A. increase the pain to a joint.
   B. decrease the circulation.
   C. reduce the patient's weight.
   D. reduce the pain caused by inflammation and congestion.

3. Cold applications cause the blood vessels to constrict, which helps to
   A. prevent or reduce swelling.
   B. prevent or reduce weight.
   C. improve cyanosis.
   D. increase bleeding.

4. The blood flow to a part becomes slower when
   A. cold is applied to a cut or wound.
   B. cold is reduced.
   C. heat is applied.
   D. heat is increased slowly.

5. Cold should never be applied to the entire body.
   A. True
   B. False
   Correct Answer: _____

6. All of the following are moist applications except
   A. a sitz bath.
   B. a soak.
   C. a compress.
   D. a heat lamp.

7. An Aquamatic K-pad has water circulating inside and it is considered to be a
    A. moist application.
    B. dry application.
    C. steam application.
    D. dry-moist application.

8. You should be sure your hands are dry before you handle electrical equipment.
    A. True
    B. False
    Correct Answer: _____

9. The part of the patient's skin that is receiving the heat or cold must be inspected often for excessive redness or grayness, indicating a burn or cyanosis, because
    A. the patient may not have feeling in the body area due to a disease process and may not realize there is a problem.
    B. this indicates the treatment is complete.
    C. your immediate supervisor wants you to do this.
    D. it makes the patient think you are doing a good job.

10. When applying the ice cap be sure the metal or plastic stopper is positioned close to the patient's body.
    A. True
    B. False
    Correct Answer: _____

COMPETENCY CHECKLIST 27: WARM AND COLD APPLICATIONS

ACTIVITY	S	U	COMMENTS
1. The student will demonstrate the correct method of heat application:			
A. Moist applications			
1. The warm compress			
2. The warm soak			
3. The commercial unit heat pack			
4. The disposable sitz bath			
5. The portable chair or built-in sitz bath			
B. Dry applications			
1. The warm-water bottle			
2. The heat lamp (perineal)			
3. The Aquamatic Hydro-thermal (K-pad)			
2. The student will demonstrate the correct method of cold application:			
A. Moist applications			
1. The cold compress			
2. The cold soak			
3. The sponge bath			
B. Dry applications			
1. The ice bag, ice cap, or ice collar			
2. The commercial unit cold pack			

CARE OF THE SURGICAL PATIENT

The following exercises will assist you to apply what you have read in Chapter 28, "Care of the Surgical Patient." For each exercise, read the objective and use information you have read in Chapter 28 to answer the questions, complete the sentences, or label the diagrams.

EXERCISE 28-1

Objective: To recognize and correctly spell words related to the care of surgical patients.

Directions: Unscramble the words in the Word List at the left. Then circle these words in the Word Search grid at the right.

Word List

1. TCIHTSEEAN _____

2. RIPSATEA _____

3. SRCTAOL PPER_____

4. GAIVNLA EPRP _____

5. GNREELA _____

6. CAOLL _____

7. PSNIAL_____

8. OMCPILTIONAC _____

Word Search

O	C	P	A	N	E	S	T	H	E	T	I	C	S	B
K	T	Q	S	C	R	O	T	A	L	P	R	E	P	D
V	B	H	P	S	H	E	A	G	L	I	M	F	I	H
E	J	Z	I	A	J	I	S	A	S	L	P	G	N	I
M	G	D	R	L	B	L	R	G	A	F	C	I	A	F
I	K	Q	A	F	O	E	D	C	I	P	K	J	L	B
U	E	Y	T	I	N	P	O	E	B	Q	A	O	K	O
D	N	S	E	E	I	L	N	K	C	D	I	D	P	G
X	V	A	G	I	N	A	L	P	R	E	P	Q	A	E
F	B	Z	J	H	O	M	H	O	L	J	M	I	H	N
L	U	C	O	M	P	L	I	C	A	T	I	O	N	K
I	J	T	D	E	C	I	K	Y	G	E	N	C	M	F
Q	P	M	R	X	P	U	T	Z	V	Q	R	S	O	A

EXERCISE 28-2

Objective: To apply what you have learned about care of the surgical patient.

Directions: Read the following riddles carefully before writing the correct answer on the blank line.

1. I carry the patient to surgery. What am I? *Hint:* After sitting for a long period of time, you may become this. _____
2. These must be measured before any surgery. What are they? *Hint:* This also describes a stop sign at a busy intersection. _____
3. This function must return to an adequate level after surgery. What is it? *Hint:* Another name for an empty space. _____

EXERCISE 28-3

Objective: To recognize the definitions of words used in care of the surgical patient.

Directions: Place the letter of the correct definition next to the matching word from the Word List.

Word List	Definitions
___ 1. local anesthetics	A. Shaving the area of the body where an operation is going to be performed in preparation for surgery.
___ 2. unconscious	B. Before surgery
___ 3. nothing by mouth (NPO)	C. An unexpected condition, such as the development of another illness in a patient who is already sick.
___ 4. anesthetic	D. Cannot eat or drink anything at all, usually past midnight the night before surgery or a procedure.
___ 5. vaginal prep	E. Unaware of the environment; occurs during sleep and in temporary episodes ranging from fainting or stupor to coma.
___ 6. scrotal prep	F. After surgery
___ 7. general anesthetics	G. Loss of feeling or sensation in a part or all of the body.
___ 8. skin prep	H. The registered nurse who assists the anesthesiologist.
___ 9. anesthesiologist	I. A drug used to produce loss of feeling.
___10. anesthesia	J. The procedure for making the patient's abdomen ready for surgery.
___11. anesthetist	K. Anesthetics that cause loss of sensation in the entire body.
___12. aspirate	L. Anesthetics that cause numbness or the loss of sensation in a part of the body.

____13. spinal anesthetics

M. The medical doctor who administers the anesthetic to the patient in the operating room.

____14. complication

N. The procedures for making the genital area of a female patient ready for surgery.

____15. abdominal prep

O. The procedures for making the genital area of a male patient ready for surgery.

____16. postoperative

P. To urinate, pass water.

____17. preoperative

Q. Anesthetics that cause a loss of feeling in a large area of the body, usually from the umbilicus down to and including the legs and feet.

____18. void

R. Material (vomitus, food, liquids) inhaled into the lungs.

EXERCISE 28-4

Objective: To apply what you have learned about preoperative documentation.

Directions: Read the situation description below and then document the findings on the sample Preoperative Checklist.

It is 7 a.m. and you have just arrived at work. The nurse gives you the preoperative checklist for Tom Green. She tells you that he is scheduled to have surgery in two hours, explains the care you are to give him, and that she would like you to fill out the portion of the checklist labeled "Morning of Surgery."

After greeting Mr. Green and introducing yourself, you measure his vital signs, height, and weight. His temperature is 100.2°F. His pulse is 68 beats per minute. His respirations are 16 times per minute. His blood pressure is 120/80. His weight is 186 pounds, and his height is 5 feet 11 inches.

He is able to bathe himself and brush his own teeth. You obtain a urine sample and send it to the lab. After his bath, he dresses in a clean hospital gown. There is no urinary drainage bag. You ask him if he is allergic or sensitive to any drugs and he answers, "None." He has no false teeth, prosthesis, nail polish, sanitary belts, makeup, hairpieces, or hair pins. He removes his wedding ring and his contact lenses, which he gives to his wife to take home.

The nurse comes in at 8 a.m. to give him his preoperative medications; the side rails are up. At 8:30 a.m., the transportation attendant arrives and takes the patient to the operating room by stretcher.

Sample Preoperative Checklist Completed by Nursing Assistant

EVENING BEFORE SURGERY

Patient's Name:_____

Identify the patient by checking his identification
    bracelet: Yes____ No____

Skin prep done by _____ at _____ P.M.

Skin prep checked by _____ at _____ P.M.

Food restrictions, if any, explained to
    the patient: Yes____ No____

"N.P.O. AFTER MIDNIGHT" sign put on
    patient's bed and explained to the patient: Yes____ No____

Enema administered by _____ at _____ P.M.

MORNING OF SURGERY:

Bath?   Yes____ No____ N/A____

Oral hygiene?   Yes____ No____ N/A____

False teeth (dentures) and removable
    bridges removed?   Yes____ No____ N/A____

Jewelry and pierced earrings removed? _____   Yes____ No____ N/A____

Hairpiece, wig, hairpins removed?   Yes____ No____ N/A____

Lipstick, makeup, and false eyelashes removed?   Yes____ No____ N/A____

Sanitary belt removed?   Yes____ No____ N/A____

Nail polish removed?   Yes____ No____ N/A____

Eyeglasses and contact lenses removed?   Yes____ No____ N/A____

Prostheses (artificial hearing aid, eye, leg,
    arm, and so forth) removed?   Yes____ No____ N/A____

All clothing removed except clean
    hospital gown?   Yes____ No____ N/A____

Patient allergic or sensitive to drugs?   Yes____ No____ N/A____

Preop urine specimen obtained and
    sent to lab?   Yes____ No____ N/A____

Urinary drainage bag emptied?   Yes____ No____ N/A____

Side rails in up position?   Yes____ No____ N/A____

Temperature _____ Pulse _____ Respiration _____

Blood pressure _____ Weight _____ lbs. Height _____ ft. _____ in.

Time patient leaves for the operating room: _____

Observations: _____

Signature:_____

EXERCISE 28-5

Objective: To recognize appropriate tasks in preparing the postoperative patient's unit.

Directions: Circle the letters of all the tasks you should do to prepare the patient's unit to receive the patient after surgery.

A. Bring the IV pole to the bedside.
B. Attach a urine drainage bag to the bed frame.
C. Strip the linen from the bed.
D. Make the operating room or surgical bed.
E. Mop the floor.
F. Place tissues and emesis basin only on the bedside table.
G. Remove the drinking water.
H. Place a clean gown at the foot of the bed.

EXERCISE 28-6

Objective: To recognize appropriate actions to take for the preoperative patient.

Directions: Decide which of the following Actions is the most appropriate for the Situation descriptions. Put the letter for that Action in the space after the Situation. More than one letter may be appropriate for each situation.

Actions
A. Listen and show interest in what the patient says.
B. Report this to your immediate supervisor.
C. Check or record this information on the preoperative checklist.

Situations
1. If you notice the patient is sneezing, sniffling, or coughing _____
2. After you post the NPO sign and explain it to the patient _____
3. After administering an enema the evening before surgery _____
4. The patient wants to talk a lot _____
5. The patient expresses concern for his family _____
6. The patient's temperature rises the evening before surgery _____
7. The patient begins to talk about the possibility of death or serious complications _____
8. You prepared the patient's skin as instructed at 7:30 p.m. _____
9. On the morning of surgery you helped the patient remove false teeth, jewelry, hairpins, and nail polish _____
10. The patient complains of chest pains _____
11. After weighing and measuring the patient _____
12. After obtaining a urine specimen _____

EXERCISE 28-7

Objective: To recognize appropriate actions to take for the postoperative patient.

Directions: Decide which of the following Actions is the most appropriate for the Situation descriptions. Put the letter for that Action in the space after the situation.

Actions

A. Signal for the nurse immediately.
B. Turn the patient.
C. Change the patient's gown and bed linens.

Situations

1. You notice that I am a patient who is bleeding and the blood is bright red. What should you do? _____

2. I am a patient who has been in the same position for two hours. What should you do for me? _____

3. I am a postoperative patient. My gown and linens have become wet. What should you do for me? _____

4. I am a postoperative patient. You just noticed a rise in my blood pressure. What should you do? _____

5. My lips and fingernails are turning very pale or blue. What should you do? _____

6. You have just measured my vital signs, and my pulse is below 60. What should you do? _____

EXERCISE 28-8

Objective: To recognize appropriate steps in assisting the patient with deep-breathing exercises.

Directions: Circle the letter of the correct response.

1. You are helping a patient with deep-breathing exercises. You have explained what you are going to do to the patient. You have pulled the curtain around the bed and offered the bedpan. What should you do next?
    A. Place the pillow on the patient's abdomen for support.
    B. Dangle the patient's legs over the side of the bed, if allowed.
    C. Identify the patient by checking the identification bracelet.

2. If the patient is not permitted to dangle his legs, what should you do?
    A. Place the patient in as much of a sitting position as possible.
    B. Do the exercises with the patient lying down.
    C. Prop the patient up with the pillows.

3. You placed a pillow on the patient's abdomen and asked him to breathe deeply ten times. What should you do while he breathes?
    A. Take care of another patient.
    B. Count his pulse.
    C. Count the respirations out loud to the patient.

EXERCISE 28-9

Objective: To apply what you have learned about care of the surgical patient.

Directions: Circle the letter next to the statement that best completes the sentence or describes the sentence as true or false. If the sentence is false, draw a line through the incorrect part of the sentence and write the correction on the blank line.

1. Preoperative patient education includes all of the following except
    A. deep-breathing and coughing exercises.
    B. leg and foot exercises.
    C. turning from side to side.
    D. self-surgical procedures.
2. Part of your job as nursing assistant is to make the patient feel
    A. lively and happy.
    B. sad and dejected.
    C. as calm and relaxed as possible.
    D. nervous and upset.
3. The preoperative patient may be worried about all of the following except
    A. fear of the known.
    B. financial concerns.
    C. family concerns.
    D. the possibility of death or serious complications.
4. One way to help reduce the patient's fears is to
    A. give him extra time and attention.
    B. ignore his childish behavior.
    C. report his fears to your team members while at lunch.
    D. tell him not to worry.
5. Preventing chest complications following surgery includes
    A. watching the patient for symptoms of respiratory infection before surgery.
    B. washing the chest with soap.
    C. shaving the chest regularly.
    D. wearing gloves at all times when doing the prep.
6. NPO means
    A. non promo otto.
    B. night procedures only.
    C. nothing by mouth.
    D. non-permanent only.

7. A sign should be posted at the nurse's station if the patient is NPO.
   A. True
   B. False
   Correct Answer: _____

8. Hair on the body is a breeding place for
   A. microorganisms.
   B. rumors.
   C. cattle.
   D. all of the above

9. It is important to measure the patient's _____ immediately after he returns to his unit after surgery.
   A. feet
   B. I.Q.
   C. height and weight
   D. vital signs

10. If the patient vomits, _____ if he is unconscious.
    A. rinse out his mouth
    B. raise the siderails immediately
    C. turn his head to one side and clear his mouth
    D. all of the above

11. If a patient appears to be unconscious he cannot hear what you are saying.
    A. True
    B. False
    Correct Answer: _____

12. It is very important that the patient void adequately within a certain period of time after surgery.
    A. True
    B. False
    Correct Answer: _____

COMPETENCY CHECKLIST 28: POSTOPERATIVE CARE

ACTIVITY	S	U	COMMENTS
1. The student will demonstrate proper procedure for skin prep:			
A. shaving the breast			
B. shaving the chest			
C. shaving the abdomen			
D. shaving an extremity			
E. shaving the back			
F. shaving the vaginal area			
G. shaving the scrotal area			
2. The student will demonstrate the proper procedure for assisting the patient with deep-breathing exercises.			

SPECIAL PROCEDURES

The following exercises will assist you to apply what you have read in Chapter 29, "Special Procedures." For each exercise, read the objective and use information you have read in Chapter 29 to answer the questions, complete the sentences, or label the diagrams.

EXERCISE 29-1

Objective: To apply what you have learned about special procedures that nursing assistants may perform while caring for patients.

Directions: Look carefully at the items shown in Figure 29-1. Label each one of them with the number of the correct word from the Word List.

Word List

1. T binder (female)
2. elastic bandage
3. breast binder
4. T binder (male)
5. straight abdominal binder
6. antiembolism elastic stocking
7. IV infusion
8. IV solution
9. IV drip chamber
10. IV tubing
11. IV insertion site
12. IV clamp
13. IV pump or controller
14. skin near IV site
15. IV pole

FIGURE 29-1

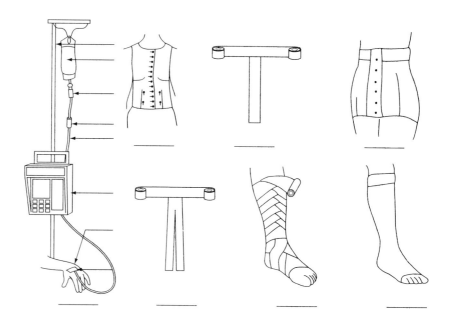

EXERCISE 29-2

Objective: To be able to recognize important safety measures related to performing special procedures.

Directions: Select the correct word(s) from the Word List to complete the sentences below.

Word List

overlap	circulation	last	size	infiltration
kinked	one-half	hour	flow rate	interrupting

1. You must provide care for the patient or change his position without _____ the flow of the IV solution.
2. Make sure the IV tubing is not _____ and that the patient is not lying on the tubing.
3. Nursing assistants do not independently adjust the _____ using the IV clamp or electronic controller.
4. An _____ of the IV solution can cause the skin near the site to become painful or swollen.
5. The following guideline would be accurate regarding the dressing of a patient with an IV: "dress the container first and undress it _____."
6. Binders, elastic bandages, and antiembolism stockings can be too tight and can reduce the patient's _____.
7. The patient's legs must be measured to be sure the antiembolism stockings are the correct _____.
8. The patient's fingers and toes should be checked each _____ for pain, numbness, cyanosis, paleness, or lack of movement if he is wearing an elastic bandage on his arms or legs.

9. When applying an elastic bandage, it is important to apply pressure evenly and with each turn to overlap the bandage _____ the width of the one before it.

10. If more than one bandage is used, _____ them to prevent slipping or uneven pressure on the body part.

EXERCISE 29-3

Objective: To recognize and correctly spell words related to special procedures.

Directions: Unscramble the words in the Word List at the left. Then circle the same words in the Word Search grid at the right.

Word List

1. RAOUSVETNIN _____

2. ISTPHBEIL _____

3. MSANMEIOBITL _____

4. CITSALE _____

5. TIONARTLIFIN _____

6. OODLB OSTCL _____

7. UBTGNI _____

8. DEELNE _____

Word Search

A	R	F	T	L	P	M	Z	N	E	E	D	L	E	T	L	S	B	C
J	H	A	R	Z	H	Q	A	X	C	A	O	R	H	F	W	Y	M	Z
B	I	E	V	E	L	D	O	Z	L	X	R	I	S	X	L	I	R	D
L	O	D	T	A	E	L	A	S	T	I	C	O	V	A	L	P	U	O
C	D	I	X	C	B	R	N	P	R	E	V	Q	B	K	G	I	G	H
K	U	N	Z	I	I	Y	T	O	I	A	L	H	P	N	O	J	B	J
D	K	T	K	N	T	Y	I	E	C	H	K	Y	I	K	Q	Z	L	E
E	B	R	I	Y	I	Z	E	I	V	Y	Z	B	E	X	A	F	O	W
E	U	A	F	X	S	C	M	L	Z	P	U	G	P	U	M	S	O	G
P	C	V	A	E	Z	O	B	L	F	T	N	Z	H	D	C	Y	D	C
L	L	E	O	Z	M	L	O	N	W	S	C	Y	A	J	P	Z	C	H
O	A	N	O	J	H	K	L	I	G	K	Z	O	W	G	K	E	L	Z
M	Y	O	T	Q	T	R	I	N	F	I	L	T	R	A	T	I	O	N
M	B	U	M	F	W	P	S	J	D	Z	F	D	X	A	V	E	T	K
O	L	S	V	D	Z	L	M	D	M	H	P	J	E	D	O	U	S	I
M	G	O	E	S	Q	R	F	V	Y	O	P	D	N	W	U	B	C	L
E	W	S	N	H	I	L	S	M	K	D	C	O	O	L	R	T	B	A

EXERCISE 29-4

Objective: To apply what you have learned about special procedures.

Directions: Circle the letter next to the statement that best completes the sentence or describes the sentence as true or false. If the sentence is false, draw a line through the incorrect part of the sentence and write the correction on the blank line.

1. Inflammation of a vein is infiltration.
   A. True
   B. False
   Correct Answer: _____

2. Binders are used to
   A. relieve diarrhea.
   B. constrict body parts.
   C. secure blood clots to prevent movement.
   D. secure a dressing in place.
3. Bandages and stockings that provide support may contain plastic.
   A. True
   B. False
   Correct Answer: _____
4. The IV container should always be held below the IV site.
   A. True
   B. False
   Correct Answer: _____
5. The amount of IV fluid that can flow into the patient's body is controlled by the nursing assistant.
   A. True
   B. False
   Correct Answer: _____

COMPETENCY CHECKLIST 29-1: APPLYING ELASTIC BANDAGES

ACTIVITY	S	U	COMMENTS
1. Student correctly demonstrates the steps involved in applying an elastic bandage:			
A. to a foot extending above the ankle.			
B. to a foot and leg, extending above the knee.			
C. to a foot and leg, extending over the entire thigh.			
D. to a leg, extending from the ankle to over the knee.			
E. to a knee.			
F. to a hand, extending over the wrist.			
G. to an arm, extending from the wrist over the elbow.			
H. to an elbow.			
I. to an entire arm from the wrist, extending over the entire upper arm.			

OTHER PATIENTS WITH SPECIAL NEEDS

The following exercises will assist you to apply what you have read in Chapter 30, "Other Patients with Special Needs." For each example, read the objective and use information you have read in Chapter 30 to answer the questions, complete the sentences, or label the diagrams.

EXERCISE 30-1

Objective: To recognize and correctly spell words related to the care of patients with special needs.

Directions: Unscramble the words in the Word List at the left. Then circle the same words in the Word Search grid at the right.

Word List

1. NCAREC _____

2. YOSOTM _____

3. EBNGIN _____

4. ASDI _____

5. BSUANCSTE BUAES _____

6. TLAENM LILESNS _____

7. SISATSATEM _____

8. PLOASNEM _____

Word Search

M	A	N	T	I	R	P	I	C	M	L	H	N	J	B
E	Y	C	Z	V	G	Q	V	K	E	S	N	E	A	F
T	Z	S	A	X	S	B	Y	U	N	J	S	O	K	G
A	H	C	A	N	C	E	R	Z	T	W	O	P	D	P
S	K	J	I	O	N	N	Y	P	A	O	S	L	I	R
T	I	Q	D	I	W	I	E	L	L	X	T	A	M	G
A	X	G	S	Z	B	G	D	C	I	K	O	S	P	A
S	Y	R	U	O	L	N	U	O	L	H	M	M	O	M
I	E	S	F	R	D	M	P	A	L	B	Y	A	K	P
S	V	L	J	H	J	X	M	G	N	J	Q	R	T	B
D	S	U	B	S	T	A	N	C	E	A	B	U	S	E
O	N	L	C	P	U	K	S	Y	S	X	S	O	H	C
A	E	T	Q	H	J	Y	B	W	S	D	N	K	I	F

EXERCISE 30-2

Objective: To demonstrate your ability to recognize the signs and symptoms of malignant tumors.

Directions: Circle the words in the Word List that are the signs and symptoms of malignant tumors.

Word List

1. A sore that does not heal
2. Weight loss
3. Unusual bleeding
4. All lumps in the breast
5. A rash that reappears
6. Change in bowel habits
7. Changes in the appearance of a mole
8. Nausea and vomiting
9. Diarrhea for 3 days
10. Unaccountable weight loss
11. A feeling of tiredness that lasts
12. Hoarseness, coughing, difficulty breathing or swallowing

EXERCISE 30-3

Objective: To recognize the definitions of words related to the special needs of patients.

Directions: Place the letter of the correct definition next to the matching word from the Word List.

Word List

____ 1. lumpectomy

____ 2. Acquired Immune Deficiency Syndrome (AIDS)

____ 3. mental illness

____ 4. substance abuse

____ 5. neoplasm
____ 6. benign (tumor)

____ 7. mastectomy

____ 8. ostomy

____ 9. orientation

Definitions

A. New growth; or tumor

B. Refers to the spreading of cancer cells through the systems of the body

C. A surgical procedure (operation) in which a new opening, called a stoma, is created in the abdomen, usually for the discharge of wastes (urine or feces) from the body

D. Collecting pouch usually attached to the skin around the stoma with adhesive

E. Removal of the entire breast

F. Removal of a small part of the breast

G. Condition caused by a virus that destroys a key part of the body's immune response system

H. Tumor that stays at its site of origin and does not usually regrow once removed

I. Refers to malignant neoplasms

_____10. immunocompromised

J. Describes the best adjustment an individual can make at a given time, based on internal and external resources

_____11. ostomy appliance

K. Means that the immune system is not functioning normally; immunocompromised and immunosuppressed mean the same and are used interchangeably

_____12. cancer

L. An individual's ability to identify who he is, where he is, and some information about time (month, year, time of day)

_____13. malignant (neoplasms)

M. Describes a number of genetically based brain diseases that interfere significantly with people's abilities to live and work

_____14. metastasis

N. The excessive use of mood-altering drugs such as alcohol, cocaine, tobacco, or caffeine that results in negative changes to one's life

_____15. mental health

O. New growths that spread, invade, and destroy organs

EXERCISE 30-4

Objective: To apply what you have learned about the special needs of patients.

Directions: Circle the letter next to the statement that best completes the sentence or describes the sentence as true or false. If the sentence is false, draw a line through the incorrect part of the sentence and write the correction on the blank line.

1. Breast cancer is one of the leading causes of death among women.
    A. True
    B. False
    Correct Answer: _____

2. The nursing assistant can help mastectomy patients by being
    A. calm and accepting of their responses.
    B. encouraging them to be happy.
    C. absent from their unit as much as possible.
    D. all of the above.

3. _____ is a leading cause of death in the United States.
    A. Alopecia
    B. Dermatitis
    C. Gastritis
    D. Cancer

4. _____ is the use of drugs to treat cancer.
   A. Manipulation
   B. Psychotherapy
   C. Canceropathy
   D. Chemotherapy

5. Normal cells are also killed during radiation treatment.
   A. True
   B. False
   Correct Answer: _____

6. Chemotherapy causes all of the following side effects except
   A. nausea.
   B. vomiting.
   C. fatigue.
   D. hair growth.

7. The cancer patient often undergoes surgical procedures that
   A. may alter the bodily functions.
   B. are not useful.
   C. may alter the form of the body.
   D. A and C

8. A surgical procedure that may be done if the colon is diseased is
   A. creation of a stoma.
   B. a stapling of the stomach.
   C. a hysterectomy.
   D. all of the above.

9. An ostomy may be permanent or temporary.
   A. True
   B. False
   Correct Answer: _____

10. Two diseases commonly treated with a stoma are
    A. AIDS and pneumocystic disease.
    B. diabetes and hypertension.
    C. inflammatory bowel disease (IBD) and Crohn's disease.
    D. diaphoresis and vertigo.

11. The nursing assistant should always report immediately if
    A. there is slight bleeding around the stoma.
    B. there is feces coming from the stoma.
    C. there is an odor coming from the stoma.
    D. there is bleeding from the stoma that doesn't stop.

12. Psychological changes that the ostomy patient may experience are all of the following except
    A. being very anxious.
    B. appearing to be depressed.
    C. being cheerful and happy at the new changes.
    D. being quiet and withdrawn.

13. Practicing with the patient to empty his ostomy bag will help him develop independence and confidence in his ability to care for it.
    A. True
    B. False
    Correct Answer: _____

14. If the patient is able, the best time to empty an ostomy bag is
    A. when the patient is on the toilet.
    B. when the patient is in bed.
    C. when the patient has visitors.
    D. when the patient is sleeping.

15. Special cells the body produces to fight bacteria and viruses are
    A. osteoclasts.
    B. immunocells.
    C. antibodies.
    D. super cells.

16. Examples of immunocompromising conditions are all of the following except
    A. diabetes.
    B. cancer.
    C. AIDS.
    D. influenza.

17. Substance abuse may be excessive use of all of the following except
    A. chocolate.
    B. alcohol.
    C. prescription drugs.
    D. controlled substances for pain relief.

18. A leading cause of automobile accidents in the United States is
    A. drinking alcohol and driving.
    B. taking illegal drugs and driving.
    C. the use of a designated driver.
    D. both A and B.

19. Drinking alcohol during pregnancy can cause a pattern of birth defects referred to as
    A. Drunk Baby Syndrome (DBS).
    B. Sad Results Syndrome (SRS).
    C. Fetal Alcohol Syndrome (FAS).
    D. Fetal Death Syndrome (FDS).

20. In situations of substance abuse, the
    A. habit frees the user.
    B. substance enhances the user.
    C. user controls the substance.
    D. habit controls the user.

COMPETENCY CHECKLIST 30: OSTOMY CARE

ACTIVITY	S	U	COMMENTS
1. The student will demonstrate the correct method for ostomy care:			
A. Emptying the ostomy pouch			
B. Changing the ostomy appliance			

NEONATAL AND PEDIATRIC CARE

The following exercises will assist you to apply what you have read in Chapter 31, "Neonatal and Pediatric Care." For each exercise, read the objective and use information you have read in Chapter 31 to answer the questions, complete the sentences, or label the diagrams.

EXERCISE 31-1

Objective: To recognize definitions of words related to neonatal and pediatric care.

Directions: Place the letter of the correct definition next to the matching word from the Word List below.

Word List	Definitions
____ 1. pediatric patient	A. Loss of body fluids
____ 2. infant	B. Difficult, infrequent defecation with passage of unduly hard and dry fecal material
____ 3. circumcise	C. A baby aged 1 month to 1 year
____ 4. diaper	D. Any patient under the age of 16 years
____ 5. dehydrate	E. Abnormally frequent discharge of fluid fecal material from the bowel
____ 6. stool	F. Washable or disposable covering applied to the perineal area for the purpose of containing stool or urine
____ 7. constipation	G. Solid waste material discharged from the body through the rectum and anus; other names include feces, excreta, excrement, bowel movement, and fecal matter
____ 8. diarrhea	H. Remove the foreskin of the penis by surgical procedure

EXERCISE 31-2

Objective: To apply what you have learned about neonatal and pediatric care.

Directions: Read the following riddles carefully before writing the correct answers.

1. When feeding the infant you look forward to this happening. What is it? *Hint:* If done in public by an adult it is rude. _____

2. You feed this to an infant. What is it? *Hint:* Many mathematical calculations are solved with this. _____

3. The appearance of this item can reveal much about the health of an infant. What is it? *Hint:* You can stand on this to reach items that are too high for you. _____

EXERCISE 31-3

Objective: To apply what you have learned about neonatal and pediatric care.

Directions: Circle the letter next to the statement that best completes the sentence or describes the sentence as true or false. If the sentence is false, draw a line through the incorrect part of the sentence and write the correction on the blank line.

1. An important part of any care given to infants and children is
   A. speed.
   B. fecal tolerance.
   C. safety measures.
   D. bowel and bladder training.
2. When feeding formula, the bottle may be propped, if the caregiver is too busy to hold the infant.
   A. True
   B. False
   Correct Answer:_____
3. Most infants eat every _____ hours on average.
   A. 12
   B. 4
   C. 2
   D. 8
4. The nursing assistant helps the mother breast-feed when he provides
   A. food and nourishment.
   B. fun and laughter.
   C. formula preparation.
   D. privacy and comfort.

5. When breast-feeding, the arm holding the baby should be
   A. supported by a pillow or folded blanket.
   B. wrapped in an ace bandage.
   C. chilled in ice water.
   D. washed thoroughly before use.

6. If the mother is sleepy, do not
   A. disturb her while holding the infant.
   B. leave her alone while she is holding the baby.
   C. worry because she can sleep and breast-feed at the same time.
   D. give her the baby until she has slept 8 hours.

7. The _____ should be notified if the mother appears to be having difficulty breast-feeding.
   A. father
   B. doctor
   C. nurse
   D. family

8. If the mother is breast-feeding in bed and appears sleepy,
   A. raise the side rails for safety and do not leave her alone.
   B. play loud music to keep her awake.
   C. remind her every 6 minutes to stay awake.
   D. turn out the lights.

9. _____ when performing infant care is important to prevent the spread of microorganisms.
   A. Application of infection control measures
   B. Frequent handwashing
   C. Avoidance of coughing and sneezing
   D. All of the above

10. If the breast tissue blocks the infant's nose when breast-feeding, he will stop feeding and let go of the breast; therefore,
    A. the mother should keep the breast tissue away from the infant's nose by pressing down on the breast in that area with her finger or thumb.
    B. she should be prepared for the infant to cry often during the time he is nursing.
    C. women with large breasts should bottle-feed.
    D. extend the feeding time by 15 minutes.

11. An important infant feeding skill for the nursing assistant to develop is
    A. changing the diaper.
    B. burping the baby.
    C. fast food delivery.
    D. a taste for formula.

12. When burping the baby, gently rub and pat
    A. the infant's feet.
    B. the infant's stomach.
    C. the mother's back.
    D. the infant's back.

13. When changing the diaper, the nursing assistant should observe the stool for
    A. at least 5 minutes after changing the diaper.
    B. color, consistency, amount, and frequency.
    C. seeds and pits.
    D. microorganisms.

14. Diarrhea can be a serious, life-threatening condition for infants.
    A. True
    B. False
    Correct Answer:_____

15. Microorganisms from spoiled formula or the contaminated hands of those who handle the infant can cause diarrhea.
    A. True
    B. False
    Correct Answer:_____

16. Cloth diapers are held in place with
    A. tabs.
    B. tape.
    C. safety pins.
    D. waterproof pants.

17. An infant with watery stools can become dehydrated
    A. in two days or less.
    B. in 2 hours.
    C. within 2 weeks.
    D. within a week.

18. When the baby has had a circumcision, the nursing assistant
    A. should check with his immediate supervisor for care instructions.
    B. should be gentle when changing diapers.
    C. should be gentle when cleaning the area.
    D. all of the above.

19. Within 5 to 10 days the umbilical cord will
    A. turn green and develop an odor.
    B. turn red and bleed.
    C. grow one inch and turn black.
    D. dry, turn black, and eventually fall off.

20. While the umbilical cord is still attached, the baby should only be given sponge baths and not immersed in water.
    A. True
    B. False
    Correct Answer:_____

21. In the home, it is important to
    A. never use heating pads on infants or children.
    B. never use blankets on babies.
    C. never use incubators.
    D. take the infant's temperature every day.

22. An infant who has not yet learned to roll over can be left lying on the couch.
    A. True
    B. False
    Correct Answer:_____

23. Keep all medications and cleaning solutions out of reach of
    A. the nurse.
    B. the child.
    C. the nursing assistant.
    D. the mother.

24. Before measuring the vital signs of children it is important that the nursing assistant
    A. check the identification band first.
    B. use the right size cuff for the blood pressure.
    C. inform the child what is going to be done.
    D. all of the above.

25. Good communication with the _____ as well as the child is an important skill for the nursing assistant to develop.
    A. family pet
    B. parents
    C. child's playmates
    D. neighbors

26. Providing good care for the child is worrisome to the family members.
    A. True
    B. False
    Correct Answer:_____

27. The nursing assistant should allow the family to help in the care of the child if possible.
    A. True
    B. False
    Correct Answer:_____

28. It is important that you report to your immediate supervisor if the family seems to be worried about
    A. a problem with the child's illness.
    B. the child's response to care received.
    C. the care the child is receiving in the hospital.
    D. all of the above.

29. Safety must always be a concern of the nursing assistant because
    A. children are unpredictable and can be easily injured.
    B. it's a nice thing to be aware of.
    C. he will be blamed if a child is injured.
    D. the nursing assistant is unpredictable and could be easily injured.

COMPETENCY CHECKLIST 31: NEONATAL AND PEDIATRIC CARE

ACTIVITY	S	U	COMMENTS
1. The student will demonstrate the correct method of:			
A. Bottle-feeding the infant			
B. Burping the infant			
1. Method A			
2. Method B			
C. Diapering the infant			
1. Disposable diaper			
2. Cloth diaper			
D. Tub bathing the infant			
2. The student will demonstrate the correct method of:			
A. Measuring the child's pulse rate			
B. Measuring the child's respiratory rate			
C. Measuring the child's blood pressure			

THE OLDER ADULT PATIENT AND LONG-TERM CARE

The following exercises will assist you to apply what you have read in Chapter 32, "The Older Adult Patient and Long-Term Care." For each example, read the objective and use information you have read in Chapter 32 to answer the questions, complete the sentences, or label the diagrams.

EXERCISE 32-1

Objective: To recognize the definitions of important diseases and conditions of the older adult.

Directions: Place the letter of the correct definition next to the matching word from the Word List.

Word List		Definitions
___ 1. cataracts	A.	Inflammation of the body joints, causing pain, swelling, loss of movement, and changes in structure.
___ 2. emphysema	B.	Engorged, blood-filled vessels around the anus or rectum.
___ 3. fractures	C.	A disturbance of the carbohydrate metabolism.
___ 4. gallstones	D.	Clouding of the lens of the eye, causing decreased vision.
___ 5. dementia	E.	Irreversible deteriorative mental state.
___ 6. hypertension	F.	Tiny bronchioles of the lungs become plugged with mucus.
___ 7. arthritis	G.	Breaks in the bones due to loss of mineralization or injury.
___ 8. diabetes	H.	Crystals that settle out of the bile stored in the gallbladder.
___ 9. hemorrhoids	I.	High blood pressure.
___10. congestive heart disease	J.	Acute inflammation or infection in the lungs.

© 1997 by Prentice Hall, Inc.

____11. varicose veins

K. A chronic disease of the central nervous system, causing tremors in the body.

____12. pneumonia

L. Type of vascular disease in which the veins are distended, especially in the legs.

____13. Parkinson's disease

M. The inability of the heart to pump out all of the blood returned to it from the veins.

____14. gastritis

N. Blood supply to the brain is reduced; also called a stroke.

____15. cerebral vascular accident (CVA)

O. Inflammation of the stomach caused by bacteria, viruses, vitamin deficiency, excessive eating, or overindulgence in alcoholic beverages.

____16. myocardial infarction (heart attack)

P. A pathological condition in which there is a thickening, hardening, and loss of elasticity of the walls of the arteries.

____17. arteriosclerosis

Q. Arteries that supply the heart muscle become blocked; the heart muscle does not receive an adequate blood supply and parts of the heart muscle die.

____18. Alzheimer's disease

R. Inability to control urination.

____19. urinary incontinence

S. A degenerative disorder that produces progressive dementia.

EXERCISE 32-2

Objective: To recognize common physical changes in older adults as they age.

Directions: Place the correct letters representing a system change next to the matching physical change.

SKS = skeletal system   MS = muscular system   RS = respiratory system
US = urinary system   CVS = cardiovascular system NS = nervous system
ES = endocrine system   IS = integumentary system   MH = mental health
GS = gastrointestinal system

Physical Change	System Change
1. Decreased ability to heal	1. _____
2. Decreased bladder tone (incontinence)	2. _____
3. Shorter memory, forgetfulness	3. _____
4. Decreasing strength	4. _____
5. Decreased muscle mass and tone	5. _____
6. Decreased lung capacity	6. _____
7. Increased pigmentation (aging spots)	7. _____
8. Increased incidence of depression	8. _____
9. Changes in sleeping patterns	9. _____
10. Decreased appetite	10. _____
11. Increased incidence of diabetes	11. _____

12. Decreased cardiac output   12. _____
13. Decreased kidney function   13. _____
14. Bones become brittle   14. _____
15. Decreased elasticity of ear drum   15. _____

EXERCISE 32-3

Objective: To apply what you have learned about the older adult and long-term care.

Directions: Circle the letter next to the statement that best completes the sentence or describes the sentence as true or false. If the sentence is false, draw a line through the incorrect part of the sentence and write the correction on the blank line.

1. Examples of meeting the older adult patient's psychosocial needs are all of the following except
   A. providing meaningful activities in which he can participate.
   B. encouraging him to do as much as he is able.
   C. showing respect for him as an individual.
   D. leaving him isolated from others for long periods of time.

2. The nursing assistant can help to keep the patient oriented by
   A. displaying a clock and calendar where he can see them easily.
   B. referencing daily events such as, "It will be lunchtime soon."
   C. telling him where he is.
   D. all of the above.

3. The spiritual needs of the patient can be met by involving the minister, priest, rabbi, or other spiritual leader in the plan of care.
   A. True
   B. False
   Correct Answer: _____

4. Patients who are disoriented
   A. have clear recall of events that recently happened.
   B. may be quite lucid.
   C. may have difficulty remembering people, places, and times.
   D. should always be physically restrained.

5. Keeping the room well lighted can reduce disorientation.
   A. True
   B. False
   Correct Answer: _____

6. An important responsibility of the health care team members is to provide safety for the older adult by all of the following except
   A. protection from overexposure to sunlight.
   B. making sure he is in a full sitting (dangling) position for a few minutes before standing up after lying in bed.
   C. keeping him closest to the nurses station for observation.
   D. leaving harmful substances or equipment within easy reach.

7. An unsteady patient may be permitted to ambulate by themselves if he is provided a walker or cane.
   A. True
   B. False
   Correct Answer: _____

8. The walker and the feet should be moving at the same time, to ensure safety for the older adult when ambulating.
   A. True
   B. False
   Correct Answer: _____

9. To make mealtime a positive experience, the nursing assistant should do all of the following except
   A. remove patient's dentures.
   B. set up the tray for the patient.
   C. do not rush if feeding the patient.
   D. identify the foods and tell visually impaired patients where to find them on the tray.

10. It is not the responsibility of the nursing assistant to be aware of what kind of special diet the patient may be required to follow.
    A. True
    B. False
    Correct Answer: _____

11. Because you will have to reposition and turn the non-ambulatory patient many times each day,
    A. you should not worry about good body mechanics.
    B. you should not ask your team members to help you.
    C. you should use a pull (turn) sheet properly to prevent damage to the patient's fragile skin.
    D. reddened areas on the patient's skin should be expected.

12. The patient should be repositioned
    A. only every 2 hours.
    B. whenever necessary to keep her in good body alignment and promote good circulation.
    C. only when awake.
    D. only when she asks to be moved.

13. Pillows should be placed behind the knees if the patient is going to be sitting for an extended period of time.
    A. True
    B. False
    Correct Answer: _____

14. A serious problem that can develop in bed-bound patients who do not move around is
    A. constipation.
    B. muscle growth and increased strength.
    C. an increased interest in food.
    D. a dangerous increase in time spent watching television.

15. As you care for the older adult, remember to treat her
    A. with dignity and respect.
    B. as you would want to be treated.
    C. with kindness and gentleness.
    D. all of the above.

16. A specialty within health care that relates to the care of older adults is
    A. pediatrics.
    B. energetics.
    C. orthopedics.
    D. geriatrics.

17. Included in patients' rights are all of the following except
    A. a choice of doctors.
    B. prompt response to reasonable requests.
    C. privacy.
    D. unreasonable treatment of caregivers.

18. According to the Omnibus Budget Reconciliation Act (OBRA), long-term care facilities must
    A. provide free care.
    B. inform the patient of his rights.
    C. discharge the patient within 7 days.
    D. all of the above.

REHABILITATION AND RETURN TO SELF-CARE

The following exercises will assist you to apply what you have read in Chapter 33, "Rehabilitation and Return to Self-Care." For each exercise, read the objective and use information you have read in Chapter 33 to answer the questions, complete the sentences, or label the diagrams.

EXERCISE 33-1

Objective: To recognize and correctly spell words related to rehabilitative care.

Directions: Unscramble the words in the Word List at the left. Then unscramble the same words in the Word Search grid at the right.

Word List

1. CATIVE _____

2. AVITONIMOT _____

3. GENRA FO NOITOM _____

4. SICOTROHT _____

5. BIMOZLTAOINI _____

6. SPASVIE _____

7. CITSILOH _____

8. IHERIABLTOATNI _____

Word Search

A	L	E	R	T	U	Y	A	Z	C	M	H	C	F	O	H	B	C
I	C	Q	Z	K	S	D	T	D	I	T	G	K	P	W	S	R	I
M	O	T	I	V	A	T	I	O	N	S	I	Z	S	O	C	E	D
J	P	A	I	C	Z	X	H	V	A	X	B	R	Z	W	A	H	S
K	G	Z	W	V	O	B	Z	V	H	Z	V	L	Z	A	P	A	K
C	Z	D	D	F	E	I	Z	S	D	Z	K	Z	R	O	V	B	R
B	O	F	S	F	U	G	R	O	P	C	Y	B	E	C	T	I	B
H	P	J	C	T	M	K	F	M	D	Q	S	D	I	Z	I	L	G
R	A	N	G	E	O	F	M	O	T	I	O	N	X	E	Y	I	S
K	S	T	Q	H	B	G	T	R	R	L	R	G	B	A	Z	T	L
L	S	A	M	X	I	A	Y	J	Z	F	T	Y	Z	F	C	A	J
D	I	J	D	U	L	Q	B	X	F	O	H	I	P	Z	O	T	B
M	V	O	S	S	I	M	B	W	B	H	O	L	I	S	T	I	C
F	E	C	G	Y	Z	O	L	B	H	D	T	K	O	D	V	O	Z
I	Q	T	A	I	A	T	G	K	O	D	I	O	I	J	M	N	D
E	P	B	H	X	T	C	P	Z	V	E	C	M	Z	C	Q	I	M
J	K	T	Y	D	I	J	Q	E	T	W	S	H	X	R	T	F	B
G	R	W	Z	Y	O	Z	C	D	Z	G	X	Y	K	S	P	K	O
B	L	X	L	Z	N	S	F	Z	K	C	O	I	D	E	O	A	J

EXERCISE 33-2

Objective: To apply what you have learned about rehabilitation and return to self-care.

Directions: Read the following riddles carefully before writing the correct answer on the blank line.

1. If your patient expresses frequent feelings of excessive tiredness and weariness, he may be showing this common symptom of depression. *Hint:* If you were in the military you would wear these items. _____

2. A stroke or trauma can cause this function of the hand to become weak. *Hint:* This can also be a stagehand in a movie production. _____

3. Before beginning bladder or bowel training, keep track of the current excretory pattern for 2–3 days by writing it in this item. *Hint:* This is also a fallen tree without branches. _____

EXERCISE 33-3

Objective: To recognize important aspects of holistic care and appropriate actions to be taken.

Directions: Place the correct letters next to the holistic need described in each situation. Then circle the best response to meet that need. More than one letter can be selected for each situation.

PH = physical needs   EM = emotional needs   SOC = social needs
EC = economic needs   SP = spiritual needs   M = mental needs
PSY = psychological needs

1. Your patient has been incontinent of urine since coming home from the hospital. _____ **What would you do?**
   A. You complain of the increasing amount of work this is for you.
   B. You encourage him to stay positive.
   C. You start a log to establish a voiding or evacuation pattern.
   D. You do both B and C.

2. Your stroke patient takes a very long time to dress himself. _____ **What would you do?**
   A. You notify the nurse.
   B. You help him so that it only takes a few minutes.
   C. You keep him in his pajamas until all other work is completed.
   D. No matter how long it takes, you let him select his own clothing and do as much of the dressing as he can.

3. Although the patient appears to receive comfort from it, you find that on days when the minister comes to see the patient, you are forced to reorganize your patient care duties to accommodate his visit. _____ **What would you do?**

   A. You speak positively of the visit both before and after it occurs.

   B. You report the minister to the nurse.

   C. You continue with your schedule while he is there.

   D. You encourage the minister to come only on days when you are not there.

4. During range of motion exercises, the patient mentions that he can't sleep at night because he is worried about his increasing health care bill. _____ **What would you do?**

   A. You notify the nurse, who can make a referral to the financial counselor.

   B. You tell him not to worry so much, and to just concentrate on the exercises.

   C. You tell him about your financial difficulties.

   D. You tell your family about his problem.

5. The child you are working with watches television all day. He will be completed with the rehabilitation program soon and will go back to school. _____ **What would you do?**

   A. You encourage him to do the homework left by the teacher.

   B. You do nothing because it is not related to patient care.

   C. You call the minister to speak to the child.

   D. You do the homework for him.

6. The elderly patient you care for has diminished speaking ability. He is understandable, but it takes him a long time to get his thoughts communicated. Today he wants to talk about his deceased wife, since this would have been their 50th wedding anniversary. _____ **What would you do?**

   A. Encourage him to talk about his wife, and spend as much time listening to him as you can spare.

   B. Remind him that he shouldn't live in the past.

   C. Refer him to the speech therapist.

   D. Continue working and hope that he will take his nap soon.

7. Mrs. Green is in rehabilitation for hand and arm injuries she received in an automobile accident. Her family lives far away, and she cannot afford to telephone them regularly. _____ **What would you do?**

   A. Tell her not to think about them.

   B. Give her crafts such as basket-weaving to occupy her mind.

   C. Offer to write short letters to her family for her, encouraging them to write.

   D. Do nothing, this is not related to her well-being.

8. Your patient spends quite a long time in bed each day and is unable to move or change position without help. _____ **What would you do?**

   A. Make sure she assists you as much as possible when repositioning her in bed.

   B. Take the time to give her backrubs twice a day.

   C. Put her body in good alignment when positioning her with pillows.

   D. All of the above.

EXERCISE 33-4

Objective: To recognize the definitions of words used in patient rehabilitation activities.

Directions: Place the letters of the correct definition next to the matching word from the Word List.

Word List

_____ 1. incontinence
_____ 2. prosthetics
_____ 3. mobilization
_____ 4. apathy
_____ 5. suppository
_____ 6. occupational therapist
_____ 7. range of motion exercises
_____ 8. holistic
_____ 9. physical therapist
_____10. rehabilitation nurse
_____11. pronation
_____12. orthotics
_____13. passive
_____14. psychosocial
_____15. active
_____16. motivation
_____17. depression

Definitions

A. Not active, but acted upon

B. A feeling of tiredness or weariness

C. Low spirits that may or may not cause a change in activity

D. Artificial limbs or substitutes for missing body parts

E. Making movable; putting into action

F. Producing, involving, or participating in activity or movement

G. The reason, desire, or purpose that causes one to do something

H. A semisolid preparation (sometimes medicated) that is inserted into the vagina or rectum

I. An approach to meeting the needs of the whole patient that comes from the belief that human beings function as complete units and cannot be treated part by part.

J. The inability to control the bowels or the bladder

K. These exercises move each muscle and joint through its full range of motion and assist the patient who is confined to exercise his muscles and joints

L. All aspects of the mind, such as feelings and thoughts

M. The science concerned with making and fitting prosthetic devices

N. Trained person who assists the patient with performing activities of daily living (ADLs)

O. All aspects of living together in a group with other human beings

P. A lack of feeling or interest in things

Q. A nurse with special training in the causes and treatment of disabilities, who is sometimes certified in his area of specialty, having the title of Certified Rehabilitation Registered Nurse (CRRN)

____18. fatigue

R. Trained person who assists the patient with activities related to motion

____19. psychological

S. To turn the palm downward.

EXERCISE 33-5

Objective: To apply what you have learned about rehabilitation and return to self-care.

Directions: Circle the letter next to the statement that best completes the sentence or describes the sentence as true or false. If the sentence is false, draw a line through the incorrect part of the sentence and write the correction on the blank line.

1. Rehabilitation takes time and patience, and it often may not
   A. do any good.
   B. bring about a complete return to normal.
   C. challenge the patient.
   D. involve the patient.
2. The nursing assistant helps the patient gain skill in
   A. becoming dependent.
   B. feeding only.
   C. dressing only.
   D. dressing, personal hygiene tasks, and feeding.
3. The child's natural curiosity can be very helpful in the rehabilitation process by
   A. keeping him uninformed.
   B. providing fear of the unknown.
   C. stopping his involvement in the process.
   D. getting him interested in his treatment.
4. Observations of the patient that should be reported to the occupational therapist are all of the following except
   A. signs of being tired.
   B. signs of pain.
   C. tolerance of each procedure.
   D. the nursing assistant's level of curiosity.
5. The nursing assistant's role in rehabilitation is to assist other team members by all of the following except
   A. listening to the patient.
   B. maintaining a safe environment.
   C. medicating the patient.
   D. observing the patient.

6. An example of the nursing assistant developing a helping relationship with the patient is to discourage him from participating in his plan of care.
   A. True
   B. False
   Correct Answer:_____

7. The nursing assistant should encourage the patient to do as many personal care tasks as he is capable of performing.
   A. True
   B. False
   Correct Answer:_____

8. Patients should be encouraged to dress in
   A. a hospital gown.
   B. the middle of the night if they are awake.
   C. the bathroom.
   D. street clothes to enhance their feelings of self-esteem.

9. The stroke patient may forget about the weakened side of his body and neglect to care for it.
   A. True
   B. False
   Correct Answer:_____

10. When dressing the patient, dress the weakest or most involved _____ first.
   A. nursing assistant
   B. family member
   C. extremity
   D. visitor

11. Transitional subacute care patients receive care that is a substitute for continued hospital stay.
   A. True
   B. False
   Correct Answer:_____

12. Chronic subacute care patients may be classified as having a high hope of ultimate recovery and functional independence.
   A. True
   B. False
   Correct Answer:_____

COMPETENCY CHECKLIST 33: REHABILITATION AND RETURN TO SELF-CARE

ACTIVITY	S	U	COMMENTS
1. Student will demonstrate the correct method of bathing the disabled patient.			
2. Student will demonstrate the correct method of dressing and grooming the patient.			
3. Student will demonstrate the correct method of feeding the disabled patient.			
4. Student will demonstrate the correct method of assisting the disabled patient with bowel and bladder training.			
5. Student will demonstrate the correct method of inserting a rectal suppository.			
6. Student will demonstrate the correct method of performing range of motion exercises.			

THE TERMINALLY ILL PATIENT AND POSTMORTEM CARE

The following exercises will assist you to apply what you have read in Chapter 34, "The Terminally Ill Patient and Postmortem Care." For each exercise, read the objective and use information you have read in Chapter 34 to answer the questions, complete the sentences, or label the diagrams.

EXERCISE 34-1

Objective: To recognize and correctly spell words related to the care of terminally ill patients and providing postmortem care.

Directions: Unscramble the words in the Word List at the left. Then circle the same words in the Word Search grid at the right.

Word List

1. SHPOCIE _____

2. LILPAAVTIE _____

3. DINLEA _____

4. GNINIAGRAB _____

5. PRDEEISNSO _____

6. CEPCAATCNE _____

7. TIRIPSAUL NEDE _____

Word Search

V	D	S	P	G	A	B	K	U	X	Q	V	I	L
F	T	D	W	X	Y	U	Y	O	M	C	T	O	T
E	H	N	O	I	S	S	E	R	P	E	D	L	Y
A	Z	O	Y	D	F	R	A	M	D	I	E	Q	R
C	Y	X	S	T	Z	I	G	Q	X	L	N	P	D
C	L	N	Q	P	A	L	L	I	A	T	I	V	E
E	U	A	O	B	I	W	F	X	S	K	A	F	F
P	D	G	Y	K	X	C	U	O	M	W	L	U	D
T	B	H	M	B	O	T	E	H	A	C	A	C	I
A	I	C	L	R	D	G	Q	L	U	E	E	M	V
N	B	A	R	G	A	I	N	I	N	G	I	O	F
C	S	P	I	R	I	T	U	A	L	N	E	E	D
E	N	V	J	V	N	E	P	D	J	C	P	K	I
A	H	D	Z	B	F	H	E	Q	N	I	G	X	M
T	Z	I	W	K	R	A	P	Z	U	B	V	A	K

EXERCISE 34-2

Objective: To apply what you have learned about care of the terminally ill patient.

Directions: Read the following riddles carefully before writing the correct answer on the blank line.

1. If you ask me I will tell you that I get more from the patients than I give. Who am I? *Hint:* Rhymes with "very dear." _____

2. I can provide cleanliness, moisture, and lubrication, and I taste good too. Who am I? *Hint:* I'm not made of only cotton like my cousin, "Q".

   _____

3. If the patient can feel clean, comfortable, and cared for he will die with this important characteristic. *Hint:* Important aspect of being human.

   _____

EXERCISE 34-3

Objective: To recognize the needs of terminally ill patients.

Directions: Place the correct letters with the matching phrases. More than one set of letters may be selected for each phrase.

PN = personal need   PON = positioning need   VN = visual need
CN = communication need   EN = elimination need   NN = nutrition need
OHN = oral hygiene need   OXN = oxygen therapy need   SN = spiritual need

1. Check nostrils for dryness and behind the ears for redness of the skin, where the tubing may cause irritation. _____

2. Learn your institution's policy concerning religious observances and requirements at the time of death. _____

3. Use a glycerine applicator for the mouth. _____

4. As the patient becomes weaker, he may require more of your help with bathing or toileting. _____

5. Change the bedding whenever necessary to keep the skin dry. _____

6. Change the patient's position at least every 2 hours. _____

7. Speak to the patient, even though he may appear unconscious. _____

8. Semisoft foods may be easier to swallow than liquids. _____

9. Adjust the light in the room to suit the patient. _____

10. Members of the nursing staff should stay calm and sympathetic when working with the patient, his family, and significant others. _____

EXERCISE 34-4

Objective: To recognize the five stages of death and dying.

Directions: Place the correct letters with the matching phrases.

D = denial   A = anger   B = bargaining
DP = depression   AC = acceptance

1. "I know now that I won't last long. Life is too short! There are so many things I wish I had done with my life. Do you have time to listen to me if I tell you a little story right now?" _____
2. "This can't be happening! The tests must be wrong. . . . I never smoked or drank in my life!" _____
3. "Well, you sure are slow today! If you take much longer with this bath I'll be dead before you finish!" _____
4. "I have prayed every day since I found out about this problem I have. I have told God that if I get through this I will devote the rest of my life to the poor and unfortunate." _____
5. "I guess this is really going to happen to me. I don't feel like talking today. I would just like to listen to the music on the radio and rest. Please close the door and pull the window shades down for me." _____

EXERCISE 34-5

Objective: To apply what you have learned about the importance of the patient's family or significant other(s).

Directions: Circle the letter next to the statement that best completes the sentence or describes the sentence as true or false. If the sentence is false, draw a line through the incorrect part of the sentence and write the correction on the blank line.

1. Members of the family should be _____ if they wish to spend increased amounts of time with the terminally ill patient.
   A. discouraged
   B. encouraged
   C. denied
   D. rescheduled
2. You can demonstrate to members of the family that the patient is well cared for by leaving the room as soon as they arrive for a visit.
   A. True
   B. False
   Correct Answer: _____
3. The family may want to stay with the patient, even if he
   A. is unconscious.
   B. is receiving care from the nursing assistant.
   C. has died.
   D. all of the above.

4. It is important that the family realize that the patient's needs are being met even though he is near death.
   A. True
   B. False
   Correct Answer: _____

5. The patient's family may ask many questions; therefore, it is important that the nursing assistant
   A. know all the answers.
   B. only answer 5 questions per day.
   C. tell them to ask the nurse.
   D. understand what kind of questions he is allowed to answer and which questions should be referred to the nurse.

6. When the patient is visited by the pastor, rabbi, minister, or other religious leader, make sure you
   A. include the visitors.
   B. provide suitable music.
   C. provide patient care.
   D. provide privacy for them.

7. Unconscious patients require more time
   A. and less thorough care.
   B. and as thorough care as conscious patients.
   C. and less work for the nursing assistant.
   D. but are more responsive than conscious patients.

8. You can help the patient's family most by maintaining a concerned and efficient approach to your work.
   A. True
   B. False
   Correct Answer: _____

9. It is appropriate to ask the family and significant other(s) to leave the room while you perform certain kinds of patient care.
   A. True
   B. False
   Correct Answer: _____

10. The patient's family should be directed to the _____ so that they do not neglect their nutritional needs if they have spent long periods of time at the hospital.
    A. chapel
    B. lounge
    C. nurse's station
    D. cafeteria

EXERCISE 34-6

Objective: To recognize the definitions of words related to the care of the terminally ill patient and postmortem care.

Directions: Place the letter of the correct definition next to the matching word from the Word List.

Word List	Definitions
___ 1. terminally ill	A. Accepting, understanding, or facing the truth or reality of the situation
___ 2. expired	B. Natural stiffening of a body and limbs shortly after death
___ 3. denial	C. A strong emotional response of displeasure, irritation, and resentment
___ 4. postmortem	D. Deceased, dead
___ 5. hospice	E. Having an illness that can be expected to lead to death, usually within a predictable time
___ 6. bargaining	F. After death
___ 7. anger	G. A key person having important meaning to the patient, and who provides key emotional and physical support
___ 8. morgue	H. Refusal to admit the truth or face reality
___ 9. rigor mortis	I. Program that allows a dying patient to remain at home or in a nonhospital environment and die there while receiving professionally supervised care
___10. acceptance	J. Trying to make a deal to change the situation
___11. depression	K. A place for temporarily keeping dead bodies for identification, autopsy, retrieval by funeral home staff, and burial
___12. significant other	L. State of sadness, grief, or low spirits that may or may not cause change of activity

EXERCISE 34-7

Objective: To recognize the body system changes that produce the signs of approaching death.

Directions: Place the correct letters with the matching phrases. More than one set of letters may be selected for each phrase.

CC = circulatory changes
RSC = respiratory system changes
MSC = muscular system changes

NSC = nervous system changes
PYC = psychological changes
EXC = excretory system changes

1. The patient's hands and feet feel cold to the touch. _____
2. The patient may speak to persons who have died. _____
3. Urine output will decrease and eventually stop. _____

4. The face will become pale. _____
5. The eyes may appear to stare blankly. _____
6. The patient may perspire heavily but feel cold. _____
7. The dying patient may feel little or no pain. _____
8. Swallowing ability decreases. _____
9. The body becomes limp. _____
10. The pulse will be irregular, weak, or very rapid. _____
11. The breathing pattern will become irregular, slower, or more difficult. _____
12. The patient may be confused or disoriented. _____

EXERCISE 34-8

Objective: To apply what you have learned about postmortem care.

Directions: Circle the letter of the correct answer for each question.

1. The body of the deceased person must be
    A. treated quickly before the family arrives.
    B. removed immediately and taken to the morgue.
    C. pronounced dead by the nurse.
    D. treated with respect.
2. After the patient has expired, _____ care is given.
    A. catheter
    B. postoperative
    C. postpartum
    D. postmortem
3. The dentures must be
    A. placed in the mouth immediately after death.
    B. discarded.
    C. placed in a bag and labeled with the patient's time of death.
    D. cleaned and stored.
4. The body should be placed in a flat, _____ position.
    A. posterior
    B. standing
    C. dignified
    D. sitting
5. At the direction of the _____, turn off the oxygen and IV.
    A. family
    B. clergy
    C. significant other
    D. nurse or doctor
6. Follow the _____ policy on care of the patient's belongings.
    A. finders keepers
    B. family
    C. sticky finger
    D. institution's specific

7. In most instances, jewelry, especially wedding rings,
   A. are removed immediately.
   B. are given to any relative present at the death.
   C. are removed by relatives as soon as death occurs.
   D. should be taped in place instead of being removed, until the surviving spouse or family makes the decision to remove it.

8. Postmortem care should be done before _____ occurs.
   A. procrastination
   B. nursing assistant resistance
   C. corpus delecti
   D. rigor mortis

9. _____ must be worn by the nursing assistant when providing postmortem care.
   A. A bath blanket
   B. Disposable shoe covers
   C. Disposable gloves
   D. A face mask

10. Cover the entire body with a clean bed sheet or blanket, except for the _____.
    A. head.
    B. feet.
    C. hands.
    D. all of the above.

11. Straighten up the room and remove any _____ before the family comes to view the body.
    A. valuables
    B. furniture
    C. emergency equipment
    D. all of the above

12. Turn off any _____ over the bed when finished with postmortem care.
    A. call lights
    B. electric blankets
    C. bright lights
    D. fans

COMPETENCY CHECKLIST 34: POSTMORTEM CARE

ACTIVITY	S	U	COMMENTS
Student will correctly demonstrate postmortem care.			

BEGINNING YOUR CAREER AS A NURSING ASSISTANT

The following exercises will assist you to apply what you have read in Chapter 35, "Beginning Your Career as a Nursing Assistant." For each exercise, read the objective and use information you have read in Chapter 35 to answer the questions, complete the sentences, or label the diagrams.

EXERCISE 35-1

Objective: To demonstrate the use of a career plan for a nursing assistant.

Directions: Label the career path drawn in Figure 35-1 with the careers in the Word List below. Next, starting with the year you will begin working as a nursing assistant, label each new job with an additional 5 years until you have completed the career path.

Word List

Food Service Worker
Laboratory Director/Manager
Advanced Nursing Assistant

Medical Assistant
Laboratory Aide
Patient Care Technician

Radiologist, MD
Registered Nurse
EKG Technician

FIGURE 35-1

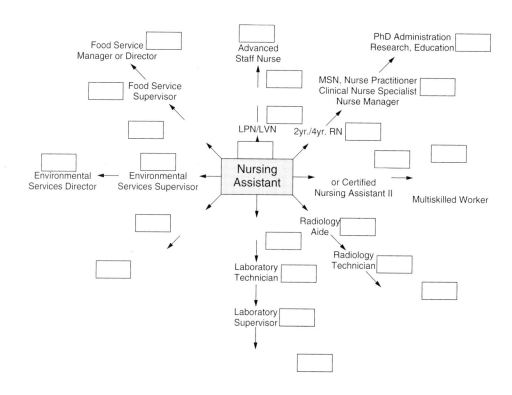

EXERCISE 35-2

Objective: To recognize the definitions of words used in beginning your career as a nursing assistant.

Directions: Draw a line from the correct word in the Word List to the matching Definition.

Word List	Definitions
staff development	Assessment of one's ability or skill to perform a given task
evaluation	Formal classes or training programs to develop new knowledge or qualify one for career advancement
continuing education	A requisite or adequate ability, knowledge, or skill
competency	On the job training or classes provided to enhance or expand an employee's skills or abilities

EXERCISE 35-3

Objective: To apply what you have learned about beginning your career as a nursing assistant.

Directions: Circle the letter next to the statement that best completes the sentence or describes the sentence as true or false. If the sentence is false, draw a line through the incorrect part of the sentence and write the correction on the blank line.

1. The Omnibus Budget Reconciliation Act of 1987 (OBRA) requires health care facilities to hire nursing assistants
   A. who hold certificates.
   B. who study hard.
   C. who hold certificates or licenses from state-approved training programs and have completed the Nursing Assistant Competency Evaluation examination.
   D. who hold up well under stress

2. Candidates for the competency examination must have completed a state-approved training course consisting of
   A. a maximum of 75 hours of hard labor.
   B. a minimum of 25 hours of classroom time.
   C. a minimum laboratory experience of 45 hours.
   D. a minimum of 75 hours of theory, lab practice, and supervised patient care.

3. The Clinical Skills Examination requires the involvement of
   A. an actor.
   B. a director.
   C. a producer.
   D. an agent.

4. Some of the tasks you may be asked to demonstrate are
   A. cooking, cleaning, and shopping.
   B. fishing, hunting, gathering.
   C. toileting, applying a safety device, and personal care.
   D. occupying a made bed.

5. This is an important time for you to
   A. ask questions.
   B. draw conclusions.
   C. offer examples.
   D. demonstrate competencies you have acquired during training.

6. After the Clinical Skills Examination, you will be asked to take a written (oral in some situations) examination consisting of
   A. 100 true or false questions.
   B. 50 or more multiple choice questions.
   C. 75 hours of written testimony.
   D. 50 open-book questions.

7. An important part of the multiple choice examination will include the use of
   A. oral responses.
   B. medical terms and abbreviations.
   C. multiplication tables.
   D. study groups.

8. Upon completing your training course, you have a _____ within which you must complete the testing process and register with the Nurse Aide Registry.
   A. "doorway to disaster"
   B. "hallway to success"
   C. "window of opportunity"
   D. "house of cards"

9. The Nurse Aide Registry keeps an official list of
   A. registered nursing assistants.
   B. missed "windows of opportunity."
   C. examination appointments.
   D. examination fees.

10. The best contacts for possible employment are
   A. local health care facilities.
   B. family and friends.
   C. Help Wanted classified advertisements in the newspaper.
   D. all of the above.

11. Most prospective employers will require that you
   A. fill out an application.
   B. work the first pay period for free.
   C. pay for an application.
   D. bring a friend to be with you during the interview.

12. You should be sure to include your _____ skills on the resume.
   A. animal
   B. dancing
   C. singing
   D. people

13. Be sure that your stated objective on the resume
   A. relates to the job for which you are applying.
   B. is clearly written.
   C. relates to the training you have received.
   D. all of the above.

14. In health care, the ability to be flexible with the hours you are willing and able to work is important to getting hired.
   A. True
   B. False
   Correct Answer: _____

15. It is important to _____ and shake the interviewer's hand when the interview is over.
    A. smile
    B. look very serious
    C. frown
    D. avoid eye contact during the interview

16. If a job is offered to you, get a written statement of what the conditions of employment are.
    A. True
    B. False

    Correct Answer: _____

17. It is preferred that you accept in writing because this gives you a chance to
    A. write a thank you note.
    B. restate the salary, hours, or shifts you will work and the date you will start the job.
    C. give a verbal reply.
    D. change the agreement to better suit your expectations.

18. After you have been hired you can expect
    A. to relax and quit learning.
    B. an orientation to the new job provided by the employer.
    C. to take a vacation immediately.
    D. to know everything about how to do your new job.

19. To make the most of your years of work in the future you should
    A. consult a psychic.
    B. create a career path to use as a guide.
    C. avoid further training.
    D. avoid change whenever possible.

20. Education or career counselors at local colleges can provide you with free information on
    A. how to advance your training.
    B. how to get funding for school.
    C. how to develop a career path.
    D. all of the above.

APPENDIX MEDICAL TERMS, ABBREVIATIONS, AND SPECIALTIES

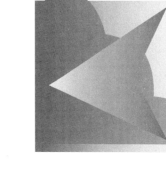

The following exercises will assist you to apply what you have read in the Appendix, "Medical Terms, Abbreviations, and Specialties." For each exercise, read the objective and use information you have read in the Appendix, "Medical Terms, Abbreviations, and Specialties," to answer the questions or complete the sentences.

EXERCISE A-1

Objective: To recognize and correctly spell commonly used abbreviations.

Directions: Define the following commonly used abbreviations:

1. w/c _____

2. s_____

3. qs _____

4. Q.I.D. _____

5. pre_____

6. per_____

7. O_2 _____

8. hypo_____

9. hr _____

10. c̄ _____

11. @ _____

12. B.I.D. _____

13. Ca_____

14. C.C.U. _____

15. amb. _____

16. C.V.A. _____

17. DX _____

18. gtt_____

19. po_____

EXERCISE A-2

Objective: To recognize the correct physician title by its definition.

Directions: Draw a line matching each physician's title with the correct definition.

Word List	Definitions
A. allergist	1. a doctor who treats patients with diseases of the heart and circulatory system
B. cardiologist	2. a doctor who treats diseases and disorders of the muscular and skeletal systems
C. gynecologist	3. a doctor who treats patients with allergies
D. orthopedist	4. a doctor who treats patients with mental disorders
E. psychiatrist	5. a doctor who treats patients with diseases of the female reproductive organs

EXERCISE A-3

Objective: To recognize the definitions of frequently used terms.

Directions: Use the words listed below to correctly fill in the blanks in the following sentences.

Word List

abbreviation	prefix	Roman numerals
medical terminology	root	suffix

1. A shortened word or phrase used to represent the complete form is a/an _____.

2. The special vocabulary used in the health care professions is referred to as _____.

3. The word element that is always added to the end of a root to change or add meaning is the _____.

4. The body or main part of a word is the _____.

5. _____ are the letters used to represent numbers in the ancient Roman system.

6. A _____ is a word element added to the beginning of a root.

EXERCISE A-4

Objective: To recognize and label Roman numerals.

Directions: Write the Roman numerals for 1 to 5.

1. _____ 4. _____
2. _____ 5. _____
3. _____

EXERCISE A-5

Objective: To recognize similarity between medical terms.

Directions: Draw a line matching word elements to their related terminology and meaning:

A. ante	1. macroscopy	a. seen **large**, as with naked eye
B. cyto	2. hypotension	b. **before** onset of fever
C. macro	3. cytogenesis	c. **low** blood pressure
D. a	4. intracranial	d. **within** the skull
E. hypo	5. antefebrile	e. production (origin) **of the cell**
F. intra	6. afebrile	f. **without** fever

EXERCISE A-6

Objective: To recognize and correctly label abbreviations of terms and the meaning of abbreviations.

Directions: Write the abbreviations for the following terms:

1. nothing by mouth _____
2. oxygen _____
3. intravenous _____
4. before surgery _____
5. every 2 hours _____

Write the meaning of the following abbreviations:

6. R.N. _____
7. Spec. _____
8. ADL _____
9. TPR _____
10. C.S.R._____

EXERCISE A-7

Objective: To learn the list of abbreviations and their meanings. This is a big list, and there is a lot of important information here. It will be easier to remember what all the different abbreviations are if you try to learn them one at a time. One easy way to learn the list is to study from flashcards. You can create your own set of flashcards by using 3 × 5 index cards. Write the abbreviation on one side and the meaning on the other side. Now you can test yourself.

Directions:

1. Arrange all the cards so the name of the abbreviation is facing up and the meaning is facing down.
2. Read the name of the first abbreviation in your stack.
3. Try to remember the meaning from studying your textbook.

4. Say the meaning out loud.

5. Turn the card over and read the meaning to see if you were right.

6. If you were correct, put the card in a pile on the left, and you are finished studying this card.

7. If you were wrong, put the card in a pile on the right, and you will study it later.

8. Repeat this for all the cards.

9. Now go back to the pile of cards on the right and study these.

10. Read each card front and back five times.

11. Close your eyes and try to say the name of the abbreviation and its meaning.

12. Open your eyes and see if you were correct.

13. Repeat this for all the cards that you originally put on the right side.

14. When you feel that you have learned them all, test yourself again.

15. Ask a friend or relative to test you by holding the first card up so you can see the abbreviation. Read the abbreviation and recite the meaning.

16. Your friend can read the meaning to know if you are correct.

17. Repeat this for all the cards.

18. Turn the stack upside down.

19. Now go through the cards and read the meaning and tell the name of the abbreviation.

20. Continue in this way over and over again, until you have learned all the abbreviations and their meanings.